THE LIFE THAT CHOSE US:

EDUCATORS WITH TOURETTE SYNDROME

THE LIFE THAT CHOSE US:
EDUCATORS WITH TOURETTE SYNDROME

JENNIFER K. STENGER, Ph.D.

JKS PRESS

SWANSEA, ILLINOIS

The Life That Chose Us:
Educators with Tourette Syndrome

By Jennifer K. Stenger, Ph.D.

ISBN-10: 0615784143

ISBN-13: 978-0615784144 (JKS Press)

Stenger, Jennifer K.

The Life That Chose Us: Educators with Tourette Syndrome

Printed in the United States of America.

To Mom and Dad and Aunt Joann, for believing in me.
Always.

TABLE OF CONTENTS

Preface

The purpose of this book is to explore how having Tourette syndrome has shaped educators' relationships in their personal and professional experiences. I completed a series of three in-depth interviews with seven educators in K-12 public schools who self-identify as an educator with Tourette syndrome. I began with a background of the participants' experiences related to having Tourette syndrome. From there, I discussed participants' experiences in regard to attaining and retaining employment. My guiding questions were how having Tourette syndrome shapes relationships with administrators, colleagues, and students and their parents. Also, I asked how Tourette syndrome has shaped their own identity. Little current research examines the experiences of teachers with disabilities. As a seasoned teacher who has Tourette syndrome, I want to document the stories of others to develop maps for career success.

CHAPTER ONE

SURVIVING WITH TOURETTE SYNDROME

Personal Orientation

I was diagnosed with Tourette syndrome when I was sixteen years old and a junior in high school. Tourette syndrome is a neurological disorder which causes a person to have movements, or tics, which can be physical (motor tics) or vocal (vocal tics). Because I have Tourette syndrome, I have been subjected to social injustice at various times in my life. Whether it has been strange looks and blatant stares I receive, or people laughing and outright mocking me or making fun of me, I have been able to witness first-hand how social injustice influences educational policy and practice. I have experienced the effects of my disability in relationship to education throughout high school, college, both undergraduate and graduate school, and in my career as a high school teacher.

Although I was not diagnosed with Tourette syndrome until I was sixteen years old, I had noticeable tics from around the age of six. My family just seemed to think that they were habits I had formed, but when they became more severe in high school, we began to look for medical answers. Throughout most of high school, I got along with relative ease. I had always been an outgoing person and was also very athletic. I was a Varsity starter on both the volleyball and basketball teams from my sophomore through senior years. My tics had also been relatively easy for me to suppress for long periods of time until my junior year of high school. It was at this point when other students started to pick on me. They wouldn't pick on me to my face, but I would catch them mocking me or laughing at me behind my back. One saving grace that I had in high school was the fact that I had a very popular older sister, just one year ahead of me in school. Because of this, although my tics got worse my junior year of high school, many people did not pick on me because they were friends with my sister.

However, after my sister graduated, more and more of my "friends" started to have less and less to do with me outside of sports. Although I was still very athletic my senior year of high school, this worked against me in some ways. I was receiving a lot of attention from the local newspaper for my success on the volleyball court, and this made one of my teammates extremely jealous. Because she was a popular girl and was upset that she was not receiving the recognition that I was receiving, she became a ringleader of sorts to start turning people against me. The last half of my senior year of high school was very hard on me, as I did not socialize outside of school with any of my classmates.

College was a fresh start for me. I attended a university with no one else from my high school except my sister, who was in her second year when I started as a freshman. We were both on the volleyball team, and this was an opportunity for me to form a close bond with a fairly large group of girls. Playing college athletics also introduced me to several other student athletes, and we tended to associate in large groups with other athletes. Once again, it did not hurt that my sister already had a large group of friends at the university, and her friends were accepting of me because I was her little sister.

Although I was having a great start to college life with forming new friends, I had to prove my competence in everything I did with respect to those who did not know me. As Douglas Massey (2007) explains in his book *Categorically Unequal*, people try to evaluate other people by making stereotypical judgments about them along basic psychological dimensions: warmth and competence. Warmth refers to how likable and approachable a person is, whereas competence refers to their ability to act efficiently and get things done (Massey, 2007). A person perceived both highly in warmth and competence is a member of the esteemed in-group (Massey, 2007). I have found that throughout my life, people who did not know me placed me in the pitied out-group. The pitied out-group is comprised of people who are viewed as high on the warmth axis but low on the competence axis (Massey, 2007). In making stereotypical judgments, people seem to think that I am likable enough but most likely not competent because I have a noticeable disability. Therefore, I have found that I continually have to prove my competence, whether it is in the academic arena with professors, in the social arena with other members of the community, or in the professional arena with the administrators and other teachers where I am employed.

I found that I had to prove myself to nearly all of my professors in my undergraduate career. All they saw was someone who would occasionally, and, at other times frequently, have strange movements, or tics, in class. During my undergraduate career, two different professors asked me to take a test out in the hallway so as to not disturb the other students. Although part of me wanted to object to this, I was also afraid of "getting on the wrong side" with my professor and was afraid my grade might suffer, so I conceded.

Towards the end of my undergraduate career, I became more open to discussing my Tourette syndrome in the classroom. In social situations, however, I still tried my best to suppress my tics and hide my condition. Although I was an English major in college, it wasn't until my senior year in 1999 that I found the power of the pen to describe and explain my Tourette. That semester, I wrote a paper in my advanced writing class about my experiences with Tourette syndrome in high school and college. My professor was so impressed with both my writing ability and my ability to express a sensitive topic with such clarity that she asked me to read it in front of the class as an example of a model paper. She gave me some time to think about it, and although I was nervous, I knew this would be a positive step for me in accepting my condition and explaining it to others at the same time. Around this same time of my college career, a close friend of mine finally discovered that I had Tourette. He asked me why I never told him before, and I explained to him that I was so self-conscious about it, and I was worried what he might think of me. I couldn't help but tear up as I told him all of this because it was always so hard for me to talk about. Alex gave me a big hug and told me that he had just recently found out about it, but the real reason he wanted to talk to me about it was because his mother was a fourth grade teacher, and that particular year she had a boy in her class with Tourette syndrome. Alex had talked with his mom about me, and she thought it would be wonderful if a young, attractive, college student would come to talk to her class about Tourette and explain the condition to her students. She also thought it would be a wonderful experience for Michael, the little boy who had Tourette. I was extremely nervous because I was not used to openly admitting to people that I had this disability. However, I was comforted in the fact that I would only be talking to young school children, and I knew that this little boy would benefit from the experience of me talking to his classmates. I was invited to the class on the day of their Halloween party, and I told them that I had Tourette syndrome, just like one of their classmates. I talked about the different conditions of Tourette and explained to the kids that you could not catch Tourette like you catch a cold. I told them that you can't get it from playing with someone who has it or from being friends with him; it is just something that some of us are born with. My friend Alex was there in the classroom as I gave my speech, and he told me that because he knew me, he could tell by the different sound of my voice that I was nervous at first, but I soon relaxed. He also told me that the little boy, Michael, beamed at me the whole time I was speaking to his class. It made me feel good that I had done something to help someone else out. It was also another big step in helping me come to terms with my own disability.

It wasn't until working on my second graduate degree in 2005 that I again found the pen as a magical device with the ability to say everything I was too ashamed to say publicly, to all but my closest friends. In one of my graduate classes, the first assignment was a self-reflection paper. It was a self-reflection with the focus on my reasons for becoming a counselor. In this paper, I discussed many things, leading up to how my disability would prove to be an asset for helping others. I discussed how I am an upbeat, positive person, and I believe attitude has to be a way of life. From my experience, every obstacle has been easier to handle when you look at things from a lighter perspective. I discussed that I handle stress by using effective time management as well as regularly participating in physical exercise.

In this paper, I also discussed how I have dealt with some trying times because I have Tourette syndrome. I stated that over the course of my high school and collegiate careers, I have become more accepting of my disability. Although I am not an overly religious person, when contemplating my Tourette syndrome, I decided that instead of always saying, "Why me?" to say, "Why not me?" I believed that God gave me Tourette syndrome because he knew I was a strong enough person to deal with the disability while continuing to be successful in everything I do. He knew I would not let Tourette beat me. He knew I was smart enough and social enough to still carry on my daily activities, make friends, and be happy. In concluding my paper, I said that I believed I understand people better because of my Tourette syndrome. I know that we all have problems in our lives and obstacles we have to overcome. I stated that I am not quick to judge other people on how they look or act, and I try to see a person for who he or she really is.

I felt as if writing this paper was a positive and pro-active move on my part. I was able to explain to my professor my disability and also let her know that it would not affect my academic performance. This paper seemed to acknowledge my acceptance of my disability.

Although my acceptance of my disability had grown tremendously since high school, I had witnessed how it affected educational practice in college. Although I was able to gain the respect of my professors and most of my peers in college, I was about to face a new arena of society that scared me to death. Entering the workforce as a high school teacher was extremely stressful for me. I was able to suppress my tics during interviews, and I always did well in interviews. However, I had two major concerns. How would my students react to my disability, and even more importantly, how would the administration and other faculty members react? With respect to my students, I knew from personal experience that high school kids could be mean, as my senior year of high school was hell for me. Luckily for me, I was a young teacher who students could relate to, and I immediately established a good rapport with my students. I am not saying that I did not have the occasional student who would make a smart comment, laugh, or mock me, but for the most part, my students have always been very accepting of me.

The administration was another concern in itself. I knew that until I had established tenure at a school, which is four consecutive years in Illinois, the administration could let me go without giving any reason. I am fully aware that it is against the law to discriminate against someone because of a disability, but when a school district does not have to give a reason as to why they are not going to rehire me, how could I prove anything? Because I was scared of losing employment, I decided at first to try to hide my disability. As one can imagine, this is not a very easy thing to do, especially when you are around the same people for seven or more hours a day, 180 days each year. Even though the majority of my students were accepting of my disability, they still talked. Word spread. Students explained it to other students, which actually worked to my benefit, but students also talked about it to other teachers. As I established close friends at work, I would talk about Tourette with them, although I never openly discussed it with many. Over time, however, I overcame my fears and discussed it with more and more people. In the fall of 2008, as I was starting my eighth year of teaching at the same high school, a former student of mine approached me. She was currently in a journalism class and had the assignment of finding and writing about someone on campus who was "newsworthy." She told her journalism teacher that she thought of me right away. To protect my privacy, she said in class, "Last year, I had a teacher with a disability, but she never let it faze her. She was my favorite teacher, and did great things in the classroom. I would like to write about her." The journalism teacher tipped me off that Kara would be coming to talk to me. She wanted to write an article about me that would appear in our school newsmagazine. This gave me a great deal of anxiety. Although it was common knowledge around the school that I had Tourette, I never openly discussed it with more than a few students over the years. I was more open to talking with the faculty and staff about my Tourette, but it still was not, and is not, easy for me. I decided that having an article published in the school newsmagazine about me and my disability would be liberating. Indeed it was. I passed out the newsmagazine to all of my five classes, and told them there was a feature story about me, and if they liked, I would sign autographs. My students were very receptive to the article. One student in my junior class, who I had had the year before as a sophomore, said to me and the class after she read the article, "Ms. Stenger, last year, the first time I saw you have a tic, it scared me because I didn't know what it was. But now, I don't even notice it anymore. I really don't. It doesn't even register to me." That made me feel so accepted and so appreciative of my students, colleagues, and employers.

At the same time (fall of 2008), I was taking a Social Contexts class while working towards my Ph.D. I had always believed I would focus my dissertation on the subjugation of women in education. It had never occurred to me to write about Tourette in an academic setting. As I got to thinking and discussing with my advisor, I realized the severe lack of knowledge out there about disabilities in education. I realized that perhaps I could make some revelations in the academic arena with a dissertation on Tourette syndrome because as they say, knowledge equals power.

As I am now in my tenth year in the same school district, it is common knowledge that I have Tourette, and I am also open to discussing it with more and more people, although it is not easy for me, even today. I have helped out quite a few students in my high school who have Tourette or who know someone with Tourette; I have also helped out other students with different disabilities.

I am proud of the fact that students know I am accepting of everyone and can come to talk with me if they have problems. I am overwhelmed by the acceptance I have received at my school district from the students, other teachers and staff, the guidance counselors, and the principals. It has never been easy for me to talk about my disability, and to be honest, I don't know if I will ever feel at total ease when discussing it. I do know that social injustice occurs in society, as well as in education. For years during my collegiate career and the beginning of my professional career, I worried about how my disability would affect the educational policy around me. I know that people are discriminated against regularly in society as well as in the educational setting because of social injustice. I believe my personality and my attitude helped me become accepted at my school district and in my community, although I know there will always be people who will discriminate against me. I believe that my disability has made me a more aware citizen and a better teacher. I try always to be fair and to see people for who they really are. I know that many people at times are quick to discriminate against someone because of race/ethnicity, gender, class, religion, sexual orientation, or disability. Because I have been a victim of this, I strive each day to be aware, open, and accepting of others, and do everything I can to discourage social injustice in educational settings.

Situated in the Scholarship

During my research on disability studies, I have come to revere Lennard Davis (2002). He is a leading theorist in disability studies, and has coined the term dismodernism, which looks at identity from a stance of the disabled body being the norm. He believes that more people will, at some point in their lives, have a disability as opposed to those who do not. Therefore, society should consider the disabled body as being the typical body. Davis (2002) educates people on the minority of disability because until more people are educated on the topic, people with disabilities will continue to be marginalized.

Anderson, Keller, and Karp (1998) have edited a text entitled *Enhancing Diversity: Educators with Disabilities*, the only book devoted solely to educators with disabilities. *Enhancing Diversity* focuses on the preparation and employment experiences of twenty-five educators with disabilities. Their case studies provide rich narratives of what the working life is like for these educators.

Another account of the experience of disability is Gina Oliva's (2002) *Alone in the Mainstream: A Deaf Woman Remembers Public School*, in which she recalls what life was like for her, as well as other Deaf students, in the public school setting. Early on, Oliva remembers feeling embarrassment for being different. I believe all people with a disability feel this way to some extent at certain times in their lives. Oliva recalls coming to dread telling other people about her disability from a very early age. I, too, felt this way with having Tourette. In fact, it is still difficult for me to disclose even today. In her book, Oliva does an excellent job differentiating between the terms solitary and solitaire. She notes that although solitary is being alone or saddened by isolation, a solitaire is a single gem set alone. She calls Deaf people solitaires in her book, meaning there is something unique and valuable about them. There is a sense of empowerment in describing someone with a disability as a solitaire. In this way, I see all people with disabilities as solitaires because they are all unique in their own way.

As I continue to research people with disabilities, inclusion is an emerging topic. The word inclusion brings to mind diversity. America is filled with diversity. Americans are all unique, and everyone needs to accept and respect each other's differences. With this being said, I would expect public schools to go out of their way to employ teachers who bring diversity to the faculty. When I say diversity, I do not mean solely racial, social, or ethnic diversity, or even sexual orientation; disability should be included under this umbrella term as well. I believe public schools, whose duty it is to teach students to accept the differences in others, should be eager to seek out teachers with disabilities who can set a positive example for students today. In my search for literature on educators with Tourette syndrome, I did not find a single article. I am hoping that this work will shed some light on the topic, and help administrators see that educators with disabilities, in this case specifically Tourette syndrome, can make a contribution to school districts. Having competent educators with disabilities makes a school district's staff more diverse. These educators can teach by example and demonstrate that people with disabilities are working, contributing members of society, just like any other minority in our country.

Questions Guiding My Research

My goal in this research was to seek answers to the following questions: How has having Tourette syndrome shaped educators' relationships in their personal and professional experiences? Some guiding questions were: How has having Tourette syndrome affected educators' relationships with their colleagues? How has having Tourette syndrome affected educators' relationships with their administrators? How has having Tourette syndrome affected educators' relationships with their students and their parents? Finally, how has Tourette shaped their own identity?

Scope of the Study

As there is no research on educators with Tourette syndrome, I am hoping to build the foundation of that knowledge base. My research is the combination of a phenomenological study and an autoethnography. Phenomenological research involves understanding what a particular experience is like for someone. An ethnography attempts to understand the interaction of an individual with others, as well as within the culture of the society where they live. An autoethnography is my own personal narrative of my life and how living with Tourette syndrome has shaped my experiences. After reading my research, my goal is for people to be able to understand what it is like to be an educator with Tourette syndrome. My study focuses on teachers in K-12 public schools throughout the United States. To participate, the educators must self-identify as an educator with Tourette syndrome. To locate participants, I used snowball sampling through word of mouth and flier distribution. I made up a flier for classmates and contacts I have within the university to distribute throughout area schools. The flier provided my name and contact information, along with a brief introduction to my study. I also distributed the flier via my neurologist to other public educators with Tourette syndrome. I also used Facebook as a form of social networking to disseminate my research information. I posted my information on the National Tourette Syndrome Association Facebook page. My research reflected the lived experiences of educators with Tourette syndrome who participated in my study; however, I cannot generalize that these experiences reflect the experiences of all educators with Tourette.

Definition of Terms

Tourette syndrome is a neurological disorder which causes a person to have movements, or tics, which can be physical (motor tics) or vocal (vocal tics*). The Diagnostic and Statistical Manual of Mental Disorders* (1994) defines it by stating, "The essential features of Tourette's Disorder are multiple motor tics and one or more vocal tics" (p. 101). Furthermore, "the disturbance causes marked distress or significant impairment in social, occupational, or other important areas of functioning" (American Psychiatric Association, 1994, p. 101). Finally, it states, "the onset of the disorder is before age 18 years" (American Psychiatric Association, 1994, p. 101).

Tics are movements, caused by a signal from the brain, to stimulate the movement. Morrison (1995) defines, "A tic is any stereotyped movement or vocalization that is nonrhythmic, repeated, stereotyped, and sudden" (p. 523). Although a person can suppress tics for a time, sometimes the movements happen so quickly that a person does not realize they have ticced until after they have done so; it is not under a person's conscious control. Ticcing is an involuntary movement. Tics wax and wane over time, and can be more prominent or less prominent in different situations. For some people, stress, anxiety, and lack of sleep make tics more prominent than usual. Tourette syndrome is 1.5 to 3 times more common in males than in females (American Psychiatric Association, 1994).

Significance of the Study

As to date, no research has been done to document the stories of educators with Tourette syndrome. There has been only minimal publication about educators with any type of disability. Only one textbook has been published to date about educators with disabilities. As an educator with Tourette myself, I want to accentuate, to administrators, other teachers, and all members of the community, that people with Tourette are hard-working, successful, and contributing members of society. They do not all seclude themselves from society, and disability does not equate with long term unemployment. In fact, educators with Tourette syndrome have something they can share. Their lived experiences can demonstrate what it is like to be a teacher faced with some obstacles in the form of their disability. Educators with this disability are as competent and as successful in their careers as are any other educators. Moreover, they can be an asset to their school districts by diversifying their faculty and acting as role models to students with disabilities.

CHAPTER TWO

DISMODERNISM AND DISABILITY

Introduction

With Individualized Educational Plans (IEPs), 504 Plans, least restrictive environments, and regular education initiative (REI) classes, school districts are taking into account and providing for all different types of students with disabilities. Ironically, school districts do not put much stock into hiring teachers with disabilities. Don't teachers prepare students for life in the real world? Aren't we supposed to set examples for being successful members of society? If students do not see adults with disabilities in the workforce, how are they to envision them as successful members of the working world? As for non-disabled students, educators teach them to be accepting of their peers with disabilities, but should we not also expose them to adults and authority figures with disabilities?

School districts actively work to uphold the IEPs and legal rights of a student with special needs. Most districts are accepting and accommodating of their special needs students. Why then, are school districts not welcoming, perhaps even recruiting, educators with disabilities as role models?

Dismodernism

Lennard J. Davis (2002) describes disability as the right to be ill or to be impaired without suffering from discrimination or oppression. Davis (2002) claims that the disability movement should be incorporated into the multicultural movement. His goal is for the category of disability to represent a civil right for all. Davis (2002) discusses how disability has not had the political backing that various other minorities and oppressed groups have received. He explains how white people have supported the cause of people of color, and straight people have accepted the cause of gay, lesbian, bisexual, and transgendered people, but not many "normal" people have supported people with disabilities. Davis believes the reason for this is that people are afraid they may one day become disabled, so they distance themselves away from disability identity out of fear. He explains, "[Disability] is the silent threat that makes folks avoid the subject, act awkwardly around people with disabilities, and consequently avoid paying attention to the current backlash against disability rights" (Davis, 2002, p. 4).

Although people are discreetly afraid of someday being disabled, it is more likely to happen than not (Longmore & Umansky, 2001). Davis (2002) notes that currently 15 to 20 percent of people in the United States have disabilities, and this does not include the baby boomers. Because of this, people with disabilities represent the largest physical minority in our country. Although the subject of disability seems to be taboo, it is not a bad thing to be disabled, but it is bad to be discriminated against, unemployed, and restricted by dire laws, architectural design, and communication (Davis, 2002).

Davis (2002) comments on how disability is a fairly recent category in politics. In the past, people did not focus on the importance of people with disabilities; instead the focus was on overcoming one's disability. People with disabilities were supposed to normalize themselves through cures or medical interventions. Davis (2002) describes the difference between impairment and disability. Impairment is physically lacking an arm or a leg. Disability is a social process which turns an impairment into a negative by erecting barriers to access. Longmore and Umansky explain, "'Disability' in other words, is not simply located in the bodies of individuals. It is a socially and culturally constructed identity. Public policy, professional practices, societal arrangements, and cultural values all shape its meaning" (2001, p. 19). It is the lack of knowledge of today's society that causes an impairment to become a disability.

Because of eugenics, the study of improving the quality of a human population by discouraging reproduction of people with disabilities, there came about a movement by the Human Genome Project to eliminate "genetic defects" (Davis, 2002). This stance is formulated on a picture of the "correct" or "real" genome being one without errors or mistakes. Eugenics is the improvement of the race by diminishing problematic people with problematic behaviors. Eugenics today is performed in one of two ways: prenatal screening and genetic engineering. Another slant on this arena is the right not to be born, an upcoming issue in courts. Basically, the courts are maintaining that parents may have aborted the children with disabilities had they known about them beforehand.

Davis (2002) wants to propose a new ethics of the body that begins with disability rather than ends with it. By looking at disability from a social model, an impairment turns in to a disability when one erects barriers or by refusing to create barrier-free environments. Because people with disabilities have been shunned, Davis (2002) has come up with the term dismodernism in order to empower the disabled. It is a novel way of rethinking about the body and identity. The dismodern era is the concept that difference is what we all have in common. Identity is not fixed but shapeable. Dependence, not individual independence, is the norm. Davis (2002) believes the new viewpoint of dismodernism could be: form follows dysfunction. He believes that we are all disabled by injustice and oppression of various kinds. He claims that what is universal in life are limitations of the body, and this is about the only thing we can justify. Dismodernism is formulated on the basis that all of us will be disabled at some point in our lives.

Davis (2002) came up with a new ethics of the dismodernist body: care of the body, care for the body, and care about the body. He explains how care of the body and for the body produce oppression, but care about the body gives us a sense of freedom. Davis (2002) believes this dismodernist way of thinking will empower people with disabilities. The dismodernist vision professes a clear mode of action. It expands the protected class to the entire population; it removes barriers and creates access for all. This is exactly what people with disabilities need. They have been a marginalized minority for so long that it is time to liberate them and empower them to the same rights and freedoms of every other citizen.

Despite the backlash to disability rights, disability studies is on the rise (Davis, 2002; Longmore & Umansky, 2001). Even though disability studies is creating a name for itself, many scholars are still reluctant to accept it. Many movies in our society serve as examples of the bitterness and resentment nondisabled people project onto people with disabilities. The frustrating aspect of the increase in publications on people with disabilities is that the majority of academics do not consider disability to be a part of their social conscience. Even though disability should be seen as a universal condition, many different multicultural groups do not want to intermix with disability. They believe categories of oppression are exclusive and should not be mixed. Although some scholars do not give credit to disability studies, disability is more the norm than not. Because people with disabilities make up 15 percent of the population and many nondisabled today will develop into the disabled of tomorrow, it is odd that people seem to be more willing to identify with the struggles of African American or gays and lesbians, each of whom encompass a smaller percentage of the total population.

Medical Model of Disability

The answer as to why people are not willing to identify with the disabled is the fact that disability troubles people who think of themselves as nondisabled. Many people work at length to be considered "normal," so much that it drives "humans into daily frenzies of consuming, reading, viewing, exercising, testing, dieting, and so on—all in pursuit of the ultimate goal of being considered normal" (Davis, 2002, p. 39). People today will go to great lengths to do what it takes to be considered "normal." For those who do have disabilities, the emphasis is placed on curing or masking their disability. Davis (2002) notes, "The medical model treats disability as a disease in need of a cure, while the rehabilitation model sees it as a body in need of repair, concealment, remediation, and supervision" (pp. 40-41). In contrast with the medical and rehabilitative models is the constructionist model. The constructionist model views disability as a social process where no intrinsic meanings attach to physical difference other than those designated by a community.

Davis (2002) describes Dr. Samuel Johnson, 18th century British writer, as a person with multiple disabilities. After citing some observations of Johnson as well as some of his disabilities, Davis (2002) notes that his tics and throat cluckings, along with other behaviors, were most likely symptoms of what is now called Tourette syndrome. Interestingly enough, although his colleagues noted his eccentricities, he was not pathologized. Many times, his ailments were not mentioned at all when discussing Dr. Johnson's character. Instead, his contemporaries tended to view him as a brilliant man with some oddities but not as a seriously disabled person. Davis (2002) believes there was a difference in the 18th century between disability and impairment. As there may have been more disabled people in this century as medicine was not advanced, people with disabilities were not seen as anything uncommon. This is most likely why those who did write about Johnson would downplay his disabilities; they were more common than today. Disability is located in the observer, not the observed. Davis (2002) believes disability is more about the viewer than about the person using a cane or a wheelchair. Therefore, Dr. Johnson was characterized by his *ability*, not his *disability*.

History of Disability in Literature

In literature, deformity is often seen as a punishment by nature. Linked to disability is an institutional, medicalized instrument to house, segregate, isolate, or fix people with disabilities. It is with this new category of disability that the concept of normality was produced. From the eighteenth century and prior to this time, there was an absence of discussion of disability. The world was comprised of many exceptional bodies. From the eighteenth century forward, we see a divided component of normal versus abnormal bodies. Those with abnormal bodies are urged to be institutionalized, treated, or cured.

Davis (2002) relates the fictional novel with the subjugation of people with disabilities. People tend to see disability as yet "another" identity to be added to the current flurry of identities. He continues discussing what needs to be done: "show how people with disabilities have been constructed historically and by and large negatively depicted by the dominant culture" (Davis, 2002, p. 85). People with disabilities in novels are often seen as either villains or innocent victims.

Davis (2002) believes others in identity politics have been wary to add disability as a member of the marginalized group because they do not want to lessen their own group's importance. Disability is seen as the identity that destroys the neatness of the categories of oppression, victim, and victimizer. Disability is seen as a less legitimate minority status than other identities. Disability is often depicted as watering down the integrity of identities. Most faculty would recommend adding an ethnic minority novel to the curriculum instead of reading a novel about disability (Davis, 2002).

People with disabilities are a significant portion of our population, and their inclusion in identity politics should be secured. In looking at novels written in the eighteenth and nineteenth centuries, no major protagonists with a physical disability were created. The reason for the hesitation in allowing disability into identity politics is because acknowledging another identity dilutes the general category of identity. Disability is still very much ignored and marginalized, even by activists in identity politics.

The word "normal" is a social convention. Normal is what society perceives normal should be. The word "normal" only appeared in English around 1850. Before then, the standard was the "ideal." In that time, no one was ideal; everyone fell somewhere below perfection. In essence, everyone was less than ideal in some way or another. Disability was not seen as the other, but simply fell on the continuum of being less than ideal.

Legal Cases Regarding Disability

In the nineteenth century, the bell curve (earlier called the normal curve) was established. Disease was defined as a lack of regulation, or an excess, that must be returned to a silent norm. Because one's social identity is determined by one's medical history, "everyone has to work hard to make it seem that they conform, and so the person with disabilities is singled out as a dramatic case of not belonging" (Davis, 2002, p. 117).

Davis (2002) next focuses on the courts and how they view people with disabilities. People with disabilities are viewed as people who believe that Nature has done them wrong and are seeking compensation because of this. Psychoanalytic theory believes people with disabilities view themselves as "exceptions" to the rule. People with disabilities are regarded as narcissists and are seen as demanding exceptions for themselves above and beyond what employers can or should provide. Legal cases have dubbed the term "bending over backwards" to portray employers who try to provide accommodations for these narcissistic people with disabilities. The courts view the people with disabilities, in these cases the plaintiffs, as bad sports, whiners, and self-centered people. That people with disabilities who stand up for themselves to protect their own rights are seen as narcissistic is infuriating. Yet the courts seem more often than not to side with employers when trying cases based on the Americans with Disabilities Act (ADA). The accommodating employer is placed in contrast with the trivializing, unproductive slacker using the ADA as a convenient cover for basic laziness.

In order to promote disability studies, one must realize that the general public is ableist (Hehir, 2005; Kumari Campbell, 2008; 2009). An ableist society is one that discriminates against people with disabilities. Advocates present disability as a social and political problem instead of a personal tragedy. They are aware, however, that the ADA will not be upheld until more citizens are educated about disability or until they are also people with disabilities. Until more people are informed on the topic of disability, those with disabilities will continue to be shunned in public and in the courtroom.

When the minorities of race and disability meet, race takes the forefront and disability takes a back seat. Women with disabilities are raped and abused more than twice as often as nondisabled women (Davis, 2002). People with disabilities report being regularly harassed verbally, physically, and sexually in public places. Cases being brought to court under the ADA are also being received negatively. Between 90 to 98 percent of discrimination cases tried under the ADA by people with disabilities have been lost in court (Davis, 2002). People who do not neatly fit into one minority status are being marginalized. Intersectionality describes the way that race dominates over the minority of disability. As Davis (2002) states, "Thus when disability meets race, disability is propelled to the margins of the class" (p. 149). Even despite activists, legislators, and scholars, disability is routinely ignored and marginalized.

Hate crimes based on disability do not carry as strict a penalty as do crimes based on race, color, religion, or national origin. Given that women with disabilities are more than twice as likely to be raped or abused, this just does not make sense to me. Intersectionality holds that when individuals fall in the middle of two categories of oppression, because they also lie in the weaker class, they are sent to the margins of the stronger class. To me, this is still oppressing the smaller minority out there. By smaller, I do not mean in number, as approximately 15 percent of Americans have a disability. However, because the United States, as a whole, is ableist, we view violence against people with disabilities as accidental, or do not care to consider that the violence brought against these people was due to their having a disability. In order for disability to be held in the same esteem as other minorities and oppressed groups, it must not be made invisible in the face of race or gender.

Developmental Disabilities

In 1973, a survey found that 750,000 American children between the ages of seven and thirteen were not attending school (Shapiro, 1993). These children were people with disabilities. Schools were turning them away on the basis that they were unable to educate them. Children with developmental disabilities like mental retardation and autism were turned away with preconceptions that they did not have the ability to learn (Shapiro, 1993). However, intellectually advanced students were also being turned away because of disabilities that made it difficult for them to speak or disabilities that made it imperative for them to use wheelchairs

(Shapiro, 1993). In 1975, the passing of the federal law, the Education for All Handicapped Children Act, granted an education to the 8 million children with disabilities in the United States (Shapiro, 1993). Students with disabilities and their families looked to the public school system for equity and social justice.

The U.S. Supreme Court guaranteed the right of all children to receive an education, no matter the extent of the disability or the cost of providing an education. In fact, it was noted by a federal court that "*all* handicapped children between the ages of three and twenty-one have the right to a free appropriate education" (Shapiro, 1993, p. 167). To counteract what was occurring previously when children with developmental disabilities were denied an education because of beliefs that they could not learn, the Education for All Handicapped Children Act acted on the principle that one cannot presume that a person with disabilities is limited in any way (Shapiro, 1993). Everyone can learn something, even with a severe or profound disability.

With the passing of this law, mainstreaming began in public schools, but before long, parents were insisting on full inclusion (Shapiro, 1993). The difference between the two is consistent engagement and interaction with nondisabled peers. Mainstreaming places students with disabilities in the same building as nondisabled students but separates them into their own special-education classroom. Full inclusion, on the other hand, places students with disabilities into the same regular-education classrooms with nondisabled peers. This enhances diversity and social justice by teaching both students with and without disabilities how to interact with each other.

Teachers with Disabilities

Christy Harrell (2007) questions whether highly qualified teachers are being passed over because they are disabled.

Harrell (2007) suggests it is shocking that school districts that have incorporated different teaching techniques and modalities to assist students with disabilities do not jump at the chance to meet the needs of a disabled teacher. She mentions that accommodating teachers seems to be a taboo topic, and it appears that the teaching profession functions within a system that does not always practice what it preaches (Harrell, 2007). Harrell concludes by arguing, "Education is a system that prides itself on preparing students with disabilities for future employment, yet it is reluctant to accommodate the needs of those who choose teaching as their choice of employment" (Harrell, 2007, para. 3).

A survey in the state of Virginia on teachers with disabilities was conducted in 2002. Initially, Virginia, as well as other states, was facing a severe teaching shortage. The idea was proposed that Virginia should focus on attracting potential teachers with disabilities in order to combat the teacher shortage. It was stated that 54 million people, or one-fifth of the population in the United States have disabilities (Jackson, 2002). Nationally, roughly 17 million people with disabilities are of working age (Jackson, 2002). In looking for information about teachers with disabilities in Virginia, it was discovered that no educational agency, organization, or college had any record of this. Therefore, the idea of a survey of teachers with disabilities came about. Jackson (2002) stated that few comprehensive studies have been done regarding the experiences, challenges, barriers, and successes of educators with disabilities. This is perhaps because many people prefer to conceal their disability, especially if they are employed.

In order to begin Jackson's survey, letters, fliers, and web site postings were sent out to increase the responses of teachers with disabilities. Larger school districts were targeted more heavily because of the presumption that educators with disabilities would be more likely to teach in larger, more metropolitan-based schools (Jackson, 2002). This was based on the idea that "schools in these larger areas would have better resources to provide accommodations for teachers with disabilities and possibly have greater acceptance of teachers with disabilities as compared to rural or smaller schools" (Jackson, 2002, p. 4). Forty-five educators with disabilities responded to the survey (Jackson, 2002). The majority of participants reported having health-related disabilities, having moderate to severe disabilities, and having been diagnosed with their disability under the age of 20 (Jackson, 2002). Besides health-related disabilities, others had learning disabilities, were deaf or hard of hearing, had orthopedic disabilities, were partially sighted or blind, and had speech impairments (Jackson, 2002). An interesting aspect of the group was that many were diagnosed with their disabilities before age 20, meaning that they received some or perhaps most of their own education as students with disabilities (Jackson, 2002). This was of interest because if Jackson (2002) could learn about their experiences as students with disabilities in teacher education programs and in securing employment, it would provide valuable information in attracting and recruiting other people with disabilities into the teaching field.

Fifty-eight percent of the respondents reported that they had their master's degrees (Jackson, 2002). Over half of the participants reported that they had been teaching for over ten years, and 27 percent had been teaching for more than 25 years (Jackson, 2002). This implies that these teachers are successful in the classroom and overcoming their disabilities. The majority of participants reported that they miss less than four days per year from school due to their disability (Jackson, 2002). Although 71 percent reported that their disability affected them while teaching, they were still able, willing, and successful at teaching (Jackson, 2002). It is possible that these educators were afraid to miss work due to their disability because of the potential for negative perception by school administrators and other teachers (Jackson, 2002). These results suggest that school administrators should not be reluctant to hire teachers with disabilities because they are afraid teachers will miss too many days of work. In fact, these teachers with disabilities miss much less work than a female teacher going on maternity leave.

Jackson (2002) stated that employers were wary about hiring teachers with disabilities because they feared the disabled employee would require expensive accommodations or modifications. However, participants noted that many of the accommodations they use are needed for everyday life and not just for teaching. On an extremely positive note, many participants reported they had won an award as a teacher, that their disability had not prevented them from achieving their full potential as a teacher, and that they related well to other teachers (Jackson, 2002). Others reported that they understood the experiences and the needs of their students with disabilities better because of their own disability. Despite all the success and positive feedback, some respondents did indicate that negative attitudes and lack of support by their colleagues and administration prevented them from advancing in their careers (Jackson, 2002). This suggests that discrimination is a problem for teachers with disabilities.

From this small survey with 45 respondents, Jackson (2002) made two strong conclusions. The first is that educators with disabilities are successful, hard-working, and dedicated professionals (Jackson, 2002). They are able to overcome or manage their disabilities, even though many of them had moderate to severe disabilities which affected them at least some of the time while they were teaching (Jackson, 2002). However, they also faced challenges and barriers while on the job (Jackson, 2002). Despite all this, these teachers were educated and successful at teaching. The second conclusion is not so positive. Discrimination of educators with disabilities does occur (Jackson, 2002). It occurs by school administration and by other teachers, and if we want to recruit more people with disabilities into the field of teaching, this discrimination needs to be eliminated.

On the opposite end of the spectrum, some of the articles I read discussed how teachers with disabilities are not a handicap. In fact, they bring a unique perspective to the classroom. One teacher who is bound to a wheelchair commented that she had an advantage on anybody who can walk because she can see what her students need, and she can see the struggles they are going to face with respect to the physical barriers in the classroom. Another teacher who is constricted to a wheelchair discusses how she can get across to students that the world is bigger than their problems. Her message is that life is full of challenges, but if you try to overcome them, you can find resources within yourself (Wills, 2007). Another success story is the one of Gary LeGates, who taught for thirty years even though he was blind. He found it very difficult to get hired in the 1970s; school administrators did not think he would be able to handle the classroom management. With a few minor accommodations, LeGates was able to be a successful and inspirational teacher. He set an example of hard work, perseverance, and scholarship. John Seaman, LeGates's principal stated, "I'm convinced that our students have gained an understanding that having an obvious handicap does not preclude someone from being a professional and an intellectual" (Wills, 2007, para. 8). Unfortunately, LeGates believes schools today are no more open to blind teachers than when he started his career in the 1970s.

Clayton E. Keller, an editor of a book about educators with disabilities, also believes school districts should be actively recruiting disabled teachers (Wills, 2007). Keller states, "If kids with disabilities don't see people with disabilities in positions of responsibility, will they think they'll ever be able to do those things?" (Wills, 2007, para. 10). Teachers with disabilities are able to set an example of success to others with disabilities, while teaching acceptance of diversity to non-disabled students.

Gretchen McKay (2001) examined teachers rising above physical problems to do classroom jobs. McKay (2001) discusses Richard Lewis, a school social worker who is completely deaf in his left ear and profoundly deaf in his right. As he is heavily reliant on lip reading, he makes sure to arrange his room to his advantage, so he can always see the face of the person talking to him. The article also talks about two teachers who teach from wheelchairs; these two ladies discuss how space is always an issue for them. All three educators face challenges in managing a classroom, but they say they do not let disabilities get in the way of doing their jobs (McKay, 2001). Richard Lewis considers his hearing impairment a blessing because it has forced him to be more visually aware (McKay, 2001).

Phyllis Seward, chairwoman of the National Education Association's Physically Challenged Caucus, writes that some administrators are reluctant to hire physically challenged teachers because of negative stereotypes (McKay, 2001). Seward also mentions despite a nationwide shortage of teachers, schools of education have not gone out of their way to recruit students with disabilities. The ADA requires employers to make accommodations for disabled employees, and these accommodations cost money. However, accommodations are actually few, and many teachers wave off any extra attention (McKay, 2001). Examples of this are as follows: One woman states, "Just because I'm in a wheelchair doesn't mean I can't do stuff for myself. I'm just a person doing a job" (McKay, 2001, para. 43). Another woman claims, "Can't is a swear word for me" (McKay, 2001, para. 44). Special education advisor Idessa Hricisak states, "They might have a physical disability, but [these teachers] don't have a handicap. These women show people that being disabled doesn't stop you from living" (McKay, 2001, para. 49). One teacher explains that working with disabilities sends the message that if you are willing to work hard, there is no challenge you cannot overcome (McKay, 2001).

Karp and Keller's article "Preparation and Employment Experiences of Educators with Disabilities" (1998) discussed the preparation and employment experiences of 25 educators with disabilities. The authors focused on participants' experiences in college as they prepared for their educational profession and also the actual experience of teaching out in the working world. The criterion of these educators was that they must have a specific disability or disabilities, and they must be in the educational profession. As Karp and Keller (1998) state, "Fourteen of the educators have physical disabilities, health impairments, or medical conditions; four have learning disabilities; four acquired brain injuries; four have visual impairments; two are hard of hearing; and one has as speech impediment (totaling more than twenty-five, as some individuals have more than one disability)" (p. 76). The authors were especially interested in how the educators' disability affected their preparation or employment experiences (Karp & Keller, 1998).

From the interviews acquired, 23 participants could clearly fulfill the responsibilities of the educational profession at some point of their career or for their entire career (Karp & Keller, 1998). Seven educators taught for more than 12 years, and three for more than 20 years (Karp & Keller, 1998). Five of the six people who were only fairly satisfied with their preparation for teaching had successes and failures in their practicum and student teaching experiences (Karp & Keller, 1998). Sometimes they received support and encouragement, yet at other times, they received active discouragement (Karp & Keller, 1998). One informant searched unsuccessfully for years to attain a teaching position and discovered that one of the letters from her university supervisor questioned her ability to teach (Karp & Keller, 1998). This form of active discouragement towards educators with disabilities has to be eliminated. Regarding support, resources, adaptations, and accommodations during their teacher preparation and in employment, fourteen individuals were satisfied with what they received (Karp & Keller, 1998). Three individuals were dissatisfied with the support; this was primarily because accommodations were not being made for the individuals (Karp & Keller, 1998).

As this study took shape, some themes formed about the participants' experiences reported in the literature. The first was stated, "Supervisors were supportive, supervisors had a narrow view and provided no assistance, and institutional resources were or were not provided" (Karp & Keller, 1998, p. 81). Another theme was that the presence or absence of support systems and conceptions about a person's disability and level of self-determination and activism affected how satisfaction was determined (Karp & Keller, 1998). Some participants were given responsibilities in the classroom and then figured out how to accomplish them. After successfully doing so and receiving praise from their supervisors, they felt pleased. Some supervisors allowed the students flexibility in how to accomplish their teaching tasks. On the other hand, there were supervisors who provided limited or no assistance. These supervisors judged the students as being unable to perform the responsibilities of teaching. Some supervisors had preconceptions about the capabilities of people with disabilities and how responsibilities of the profession must be accomplished (Karp & Keller, 1998).

Besides supervisors, active support systems proved to be significant in the participant's lives. The support systems contributed to the individuals' self-worth and ability to continue on in the profession even in the face of adversity (Karp & Keller, 1998). One woman's parents played a significant role in developing her sense of independence and her ability to achieve her career goals (Karp & Keller, 1998). Another woman's dysfunctional family did not have high expectations for her, but two of her elementary teachers helped her realize her potential and reinforced her strengths (Karp & Keller, 1998). Support systems can also come by way of financial assistance and professional support groups. Four individuals received financial aid to attend college from state vocational rehabilitation agencies (Karp & Keller, 1998).

Perhaps even stronger than support systems is each individual's own self-concept, self-determination, and disability activism. One woman did not see herself as disabled, but as someone who has difficulty carrying things. Another woman believed her knowledge of her disability and its effects helped her in her teaching. One man was denied admission to a master's program because of his disability, with the rejection letter stating the campus was not accessible for him. Another woman received no accommodations during college and was questioned about how she thought she could become a teacher. She found a way around student teaching by being accepted into graduate school and using her paraprofessional experience to replace student teaching (Karp & Keller, 1998). She now uses her knowledge about Section 504 to educate her school administrators and officials in her teachers' union (Karp & Keller, 1998). She has become an advocate for herself and other individuals with disabilities.

In conclusion of this study, almost all of the educators with disabilities could satisfactorily perform the responsibilities of their profession for at least part, if not all, of their careers (Karp & Keller, 1998). They used adaptations, accommodations, and resources provided by their universities, school districts, colleagues, students, and themselves to fulfill the requirements of their teaching experience. When the individuals with disabilities in the study were judged unsatisfactory in their performance, there seemed to be preconceptions about the educators' capabilities. Karp and Keller (1998) state that, "[This shows] that the perspectives and actions of preparation personnel, supervisors, and administrators can greatly affect the performance and success of educators with disabilities" (p. 85). In short, teachers, administrators, parents, and university faculty can either foster or hinder an individual's development as a teacher.

Attitudes Towards Educators with Disabilities

Karp and Keller (1998) provide challenges to the field of education. One deals with adjusting the ways in which we view the career development and process of becoming an educator (Karp & Keller, 1998). Instead of focusing on particular behaviors or specific tasks that must be performed, there needs to be more of a focus on the competencies of educational professionals. This may expand the possibilities for people with disabilities. Another challenge involves expanding our ideas about the place of a disability in a person's life. Karp and Keller (1998) state, "It is important for university faculty and school district administrators not to assume or predetermine how an educator with a disability acknowledges his or her disability, defines it, copes with it, adapts to it, and internalizes it into his or her self-concept" (p. 85). Administrators also need to be willing to see the capabilities, not the difficulties, in individuals with disabilities, and view them as possible candidates for educational professions (Karp & Keller, 1998).

The article "Attitudes toward Teachers with Disabilities" (1998) also discussed attitudes towards educators with disabilities. It has been pointed out that negative attitudes toward persons with disabilities appear to be influenced by a country's economic, social, and cultural status (Anderson, 1998). It is also noted that the attitudes of nondisabled people toward persons with disabilities can and do have a tremendous influence on the quality of life of persons with disabilities (Anderson, 1998). Although no records have been kept on people with disabilities from early history, archeological studies suggest that people with disabilities existed more than forty-five thousand years ago (Anderson, 1998). In many early cultures, these people were treated with brutality, prejudice, and neglect, and religious teachings suggested that disabilities were a consequence of sinful behavior or the lack of faith in God on the part of the person with a disability or his or her parents (Anderson, 1998).

There is little research on the attitudes professors hold toward students with disabilities. What does exist suggests that most professors have fairly favorable attitudes toward students with disabilities on campus, although attitudes are less positive about having students with disabilities in their own department (Anderson, 1998). It has been noted that programs that welcome students with disabilities often have professors who have had experience with students with disabilities. Ironically enough, some professors in special education, who should have had training in adapting programs for students with disabilities, do not know how to accommodate a student with a disability. Anderson (1998) states, "Lack of communication, fear, and lack of understanding all contribute to discriminatory behaviors directed at students with disabilities" (p. 185). Today, many universities have an office of disability support services designed to provide support services for students with disabilities. These services may include tutoring, mobility training, personal counseling, or intervention with instructors if the student is not successful in receiving accommodations.

For college students in teacher preparation programs, they may face obstacles such as inaccessible school buildings, inadequate parking, unusable rest room facilities, and negative attitudes of school administrators (Anderson, 1998). All of this can create difficulties for job applicants with a disability. The Rehabilitation Act, Section 504, and the Americans with Disabilities Act prohibit discrimination on the basis of disability; however, the act states that accommodations should not cause an "undue hardship" on any agency or business (Anderson, 1998, p. 186). Anderson (1998) states, "[As for actual employment,] the attitudes of administrators and human resource personnel toward persons with disabilities are influenced by a number of factors, including previous contact or experience with employees who have disabilities, the type and severity of disability, responsibility for the disability, the visibility of the disability, the nature of the specific job for which the person is applying, and the degree of exposure that persons with disabilities have with the public" (pp. 186-7). Employers expressed more concern the more visible the disability. Employers also stated the most important factors regarding the decision to hire people with disabilities are the ability to perform the job, productivity, compliance with affirmative action, absenteeism, and positive public relations (Anderson, 1998). Although there is little research concerning the attitudes of school administrators, it has been indicated that the administrators showed discrimination in their hiring practices (Anderson, 1998). It has also been noted that younger administrators are more willing to hire applicants with disabilities than older administrators (Anderson, 1998).

Many persons with disabilities who were encouraged to enter the education profession were pressured to major in special education. These people reported that career counselors believed educators with disabilities could not teach in the regular classroom (Anderson, 1998). Anderson (1998) states, "Decisions about the ability to teach should be based on practical experience and not on the perceptions of career counselors or professors" (p. 189).

Another problem individuals with disabilities who wish to teach may encounter is state regulations requiring that applicants must be free of disqualifying physical, mental, or emotional disability. Anderson (1998) notes, "[The problem with this is that the decision of] what constitutes a disqualifying disability is left to physicians who have little knowledge about job requirements in a school classroom or about the type of accommodations that can be provided for specific disabilities" (p. 189). Other reasons cited by school administrators for not employing persons with disabilities are safety issues and insurance concerns. Accessibility was cited as a major reason for not finding employment by people with disabilities.

Anderson (1998) notes, "[Currently,] little information is available about (*a*) the number of people with disabilities who are choosing education as a career choice, (*b*) accommodations and support services that are needed to assist students with disabilities in preparation programs and practica experiences, and (*c*) the number of people with disabilities who become employed with the public schools" (p. 189). Even without this information, individuals with the ability, desire, knowledge, and skill should not be discouraged or prevented from obtaining a teaching certificate or from becoming a classroom teacher; they should be encouraged (Anderson, 1998).

In conclusion, it is apparent that although there may be some speculation by university supervisors and school district administrators, individuals with disabilities have the competence to perform the duties of a professional educator, and do so with success. Until both universities and school districts actively recruit professional educators with disabilities, public education will be missing a fundamental aspect of American diversity. Public education is adamant about upholding Individualized Education Plans and all types of Individualized Education's practices and policies. However, until students see teachers with disabilities successfully holding down teaching positions, how will we ever teach our students to accept diversity of all kinds?

Disability As a Minority

Educators with disabilities are a silent and often invisible minority that society knows very little about. Brock (2007) stated that research has mainly focused on pre-service teachers with disabilities studying to be teachers but not that of educators with disabilities working in school organizations. Brock (2007) notes this lack of knowledge and research is both surprising and concerning because the number of educators with disabilities is growing and will most likely continue to grow.

Brock (2007) discussed that the limited body of knowledge on educators with disabilities may stem from the fact that individuals are reluctant to disclose disabilities. The number of educators who gave good reasons for doing just this saddened me. The article states the American with Disabilities Act (ADA) of 1990 and Section 504 of the Rehabilitation Act of 1993 mandate equal employment practices for individuals with disabilities (Brock, 2007). Brock (2007) even defines a disability, which, "According to the ADA, a person who has a physical or mental impairment that substantially limits one or more life activities or a person who has a record of such impairments is considered to have a disability" (p. 9). However, even with the passing of these two important acts, the employment rate of people with disabilities has only grown slightly (Brock, 2007). It gets worse. At one point Brock (2007) stated, "In some instances, the law's complexity may have worsened employment opportunities due to employers' fears of incurring costs related to providing accommodations" (p. 9).

From there, Brock (2007) moves to her study, in which she studied a small but wide range of educators. She first selected 12 participants, but two did not participate in the study due to time constraints (Brock, 2007). Of the ten educators who did participate in her study, eight of the ten had illnesses that surfaced mid-career. Of the ten educators, two were elementary principals, one an elementary teacher, two high school teachers, four college professors, and one a college administrator (Brock, 2007). The interview questions Brock (2007) used were based on "items on social treatment, architectural barriers, workplace accommodations, revelation of disability, productivity, and career mobility" (p. 10).

One section of Brock's (2007) article that inspired me, instead of depressing me, was when the participants talked about their educational attainment. Seven of the participants had master's degrees in education; one had two master's degrees; and two had doctorates (Brock, 2007). This inspired me to see that other people with disabilities, besides myself, work to continue their education.

Participants revealed that "disabilities often were viewed as a source of social discrimination; architectural barriers frequently presented obstacles; accommodations were minimal; invisible disabilities were usually concealed; disabilities prompted overwork; and disabilities limited career mobility in some cases" (Brock, 2007, p. 10). The main differences in responses were from educators with visible and invisible disabilities. Seven of the ten participants reported incidents of disability-related social discrimination in their workplace (Brock, 2007). One participant explained that the stigma for people with disabilities is a sign that you are damaged goods (Brock, 2007). Another educator observed that although there are fewer barriers today than in the past, social barriers remain.

Prejudice is not easily overcome. It may not be right, but it is a fact. In discussing accommodations, seven of the participants reported that they avoided asking for accommodations (Brock, 2007). Several respondents chose to provide their own. One quote that disheartened me was when a college professor stated, "Generally, if you can find a way to work around the situation, it's probably easier to do it. A simple fact of life with a disability is that often a request for help causes more problems than you started with" (Brock, 2007, p. 11). Another sad quote was from a college administrator who said, "My advice for others is to do whatever you can for yourself— quietly. Don't ask for anything" (Brock, 2007, p. 11). This is so upsetting because it makes me wonder what was the purpose for passing ADA or Section 504 if workers with a disability cannot ask for reasonable accommodations.

Ableism and Disablism

To disclose or conceal one's disability may be determined because of ableism and disablism. Ableism is defined as the discrimination against disabled people (Hehir, 2005; Kumari Campbell, 2008; 2009). Kumari Campbell gives a definition of disablism, as it is not the same as ableism. She claims, "Disablism is a set of assumptions and practices promoting the differential or unequal treatment of people because of actual or presumed disabilities" (Kumari Campbell, 2008, p. 152). For instance, some people are openly shocked when I mention past boyfriends or when I tell them I am going on a date. I am subjected to disablism because of their stereotypical judgments that a woman with Tourette is not able to be romantically involved with someone. I have experienced disablism not only in my personal life but in my academic life as well. Throughout my college education, both graduate and undergraduate, I have had to prove my academic worth to my professors. With no prior knowledge of my abilities, I was just another name on a roster. Actually, I was worse. I was "that student." I would venture that all my professors knew my name, or at least remembered me, after our initial class session. I was that girl who jerked her neck or her arms; I was that girl who kept clapping her hands in class. I was that girl no one could understand.

Because of disablism, no one assumed that I could be intelligent. Who would have thought that such a girl would have one of the highest grades in the class? I will never forget getting back a calculus exam my freshman year of college. My professor wrote at the top, "98%, the highest grade in the class. Now to get you to stop hitting yourself in the head!" I know she was not making fun of me. I honestly believe that she just did not understand me.

Although disablism seems very similar to ableism, Kumari Campbell (2008) explains their differences. She comments, "Disablism relates to the production of disability and fits well into a social constructionist understanding of disability. Whereas ableism can be associated with the production of ableness, the perfectible body and, by default, the creation of a neologism that suggests a falling away from ableness that is disability" (Kumari Campbell, 2008, pp. 152-3). Disablism is a result of not understanding something, and therefore believing one's preconceived stereotypical assumptions that a person with a disability is not as competent as a non-disabled person. Ableism is the direct discrimination of someone for having a disability. Disablism occurs because of a lack of knowledge; one does not know any better. An ableist is aware of what he is doing; he believes he is better than a person with a disability because he is non-disabled. Kumari Campbell continues, "As a conceptual tool ableism transcends levels of governance related to the procedures, structure, institutions and values of civil society and locates itself clearly in the arena of genealogies of knowledge. Ableism is deeply and subliminally embedded within our culture" (Kumari Campbell, 2008, p.

153). As a person with a disability, I would completely agree with that statement. People with disabilities face discrimination in many, if not all, of the places they go in public.

Kumari Campbell (2008) goes on to explain that the process of ableism sees "perfected" people as preferable. A chief belief of ableists is that if possible, the disability or disabled person should "be ameliorated, cured or indeed eliminated" (p. 154). Kumari Campbell (2008) then moves on to discuss internalized ableism, or internalized oppression. Rosenwasser (2000) defined internalized oppression by stating, "[It is] an involuntary reaction to oppression which originates outside one's group and which results in group members loathing themselves, disliking others in their group, and blaming themselves for the oppression—rather than realizing that these beliefs are constructed in them by oppressive socio-economic political systems" (p. 1). Although this saddens me, I can relate to it well. I can clearly recall times when I felt like less of a person, less of a woman, less of a citizen, and hated myself for having this disability that made me an outcast in my high school. Kumari Campbell (2008) describes how internalized ableism is basically disabled self-hatred. Internalized ableism mutes a person with a disability for asking for help or even for advocating for herself. I can also relate to this because as an educator, I was worried about disclosing my disability for fear of keeping a job and attaining tenure status. Therefore, I was left on my own to deal with all the challenges and demands of being a new teacher, all the while trying to mask the symptoms of my disability, which only succeeded in adding more stress and pressure to my performance.

Conclusion

Clearly, many people with disabilities believe they need to hide their disability or distance themselves from others simply to keep the peace. This is internalized ableism; it is when people with disabilities truly believe something is wrong with them for being the way they are. Therefore, they end up hating themselves for having the disability—something they did not elect to have in the first place. In Oliva's (2004) research, one participant stated, "I felt like I was a burden to others, so I felt it wise to keep a distance. This didn't seem to bother anyone— no one reached out to me" (p. 82). Many participants did not want to call unwanted attention to their "differences." Unfortunately, Oliva (2004) and her participants mentioned that it is possible for children with disabilities to focus solely on their studies and forego friendship entirely.

Conforming to ableism by hiding their disability in order to appear normal is one of the factors that creates internalized ableism. By trying to conform, people with disabilities end up loathing themselves for having the disability and not being "normal" in the first place. Deborah Marks (1999) states, "Internalized oppression is not the cause of our mistreatment; it is the result of our mistreatment. It would not exist without the real external oppression that forms the social climate in which we exist. Once oppression has been internalized, little force is needed to keep us submissive. We harbor inside ourselves the pain and the memories, the fears and the confusions, the negative self-images and the low expectations, turning them into weapons with which to re-injure ourselves, every day of our lives" (p. 25). This quote truly is what a person with a disability lives through day after day.

CHAPTER THREE

HOW I WENT ABOUT MY STUDY

Overview

This chapter covers the methodology of my research. It includes the design of the study, the role of the researcher, the limitations of the study, a description of the participants, the data collection, and data analysis. The purpose of this study is to explore the experiences of educators with Tourette syndrome, particularly the experiences that relate to interaction with administrators, other faculty, and students and their parents. This study seeks to understand how having Tourette syndrome has shaped educators' relationships in their personal and professional experiences. The goal is to develop a theoretical framework around stronger support and value for teachers with disabilities, particularly with visible behaviors such as Tourette syndrome.

Design of Study

The design of this qualitative study is both phenomenological and autoethnographic. I chose to perform a qualitative study because qualitative research attempts to understand processes, concepts, and ideas, and it is not measured in numbers. Qualitative research focuses on how people interpret their experiences, how they construct their lives, and the meanings they attach to their experiences (Merriam, 2009). Merriam (2009) states, "The overall purpose is to *understand* how people make sense of their lives and their experiences" (p. 23).

My qualitative study was phenomenological, in that through my research, a reader will be able to better understand what life is like for an educator with Tourette syndrome. Phenomenological research involves knowing what a life experience was like for someone else. It is being able to say, "I understand what this person went through." Oliva (2004) explains that in a phenomenological study, a researcher is not looking for cause and effect relationships, but looking to tell the story of the people who have lived through a particular experience. Merriam (2009) describes phenomenological research as "a focus on the experience itself and how that experience is transformed into consciousness" (p. 24). I want my readers to be able to understand what my participants went through because not a lot of people know about or can relate to Tourette syndrome. I believe other educators and administrators can learn what it is like to be an educator with Tourette syndrome and how this disability has affected one's private life, as well as one's professional life in dealing with students, their parents, colleagues, and administrators. Phenomenological research can go a long way in terms of teaching people about areas of life they otherwise would have no experience with or knowledge about. I want more people to know about Tourette syndrome and to be able to better understand people with a disability, and phenomenological research will be key in this process.

My study was also autoethnographic, as I incorporated my own personal story and experiences I have had as both a student and an educator with Tourette syndrome. An autoethnography is material you believe others will want to know about, as depicted through your eyes and direct experience (Wolcott, 2010). Merriam (2009) explains ethnography as research that attempts to understand the interaction of individuals not only with others, but also within the culture of the society where they live. Therefore, an autoethnography is the study of my own life and how living with Tourette syndrome has shaped my personal experiences.

In conducting phenomenological research, the interview is the chief technique of data collection (Merriam, 2009). Patton (2002) states that the purpose of interviewing is to allow the researcher into the participant's perspective. I relied heavily on Seidman's (2006) in-depth interview technique. Seidman (2006) states, "Telling stories is essentially a meaning-making process" (p. 7). He explains further, "At the root of in-depth interviewing is an interest in understanding the lived experiences of other people and the meaning they make of that experience" (Seidman, 2006, p. 9). The three-interview structure is a phenomenological approach. In the first interview, the context of the participant's experience is established. The second interview allows the participant to reconstruct his experience, and the third interview prompts the participant to reflect on the meaning that this experience holds for her personally.

The first interview is started by asking the participant to tell you as much about himself or herself as possible up to the present time. In short, the researcher is asking for one's life history. The participant is asked to reconstruct his experiences with family, school, friends, neighborhood, and work (Seidman, 2006). In essence, the participant is telling us the narrative of her life. Merriam (2009) explains, "Stories, also called 'narratives' have become a popular source of data in qualitative research. The key to this type of qualitative research is the use of stories as data, and more specifically, first-person accounts of experience told in story form having a beginning, middle, and end" (p. 32). The second interview concentrates on the concrete details of the participant's present lived experiences as they relate to the topic (Seidman, 2006). You may ask a teacher what a typical day teaching is like for her from the time she wakes up to the time she falls asleep. In the third interview, the participant is asked to reflect on the meaning of that experience. By asking the question of "meaning," it "addresses the intellectual and emotional connections between the participant's life and work" (Seidman, 2006, p. 18).

Role of Researcher

My role as an educator with Tourette syndrome was reflected on heavily before, during, and after my research was conducted. I disclosed my identity as an educator with Tourette syndrome in the initial contact with each participant. As I coded each transcript, I was cognizant that my identity as an educator with Tourette syndrome did not lead me to believe certain implications in participants' responses and stories. I was also aware that I actively listened to my participants' stories without projecting my stories onto them.

Limitations of Study

One limitation of my study was that the size of the study was small, as I only interviewed seven participants. However, I reached saturation of information by interviewing my seven participants. Although my study reflected the thoughts and perceptions of educators with Tourette syndrome, I cannot generalize that these perceptions are the same for all educators with Tourette syndrome. Another limitation that has to be considered is that the participants may have been nervous and cautious about what they disclosed regarding administrators from their school district. Even though identities have been kept confidential, participants may have been cautious, as there are not a great number of educators with Tourette syndrome, so they may have been worried about repercussions in district if they were critical.

Participation in this study was voluntary. I reached participants through snowball sampling. I disseminated fliers about the purpose of the study, along with my contact information, throughout school districts in the nation by means of email forwarding and listservs. I also posted my research plans on the National Tourette Syndrome Association Facebook page. They have over 8,000 fans, and I was able to enlist some participants via this form of social networking.

The participants contacted me via home phone, cell phone, or email; I did not breech anyone's identity by asking people to provide me names of possible participants.

Participants

Before conducting my research, I was aware that my largest challenge would be locating participants. I was not sure of how many educators with Tourette syndrome I would be able to locate. I hoped that these educators would be eager to share their stories with me. I hoped that this study would give educators with Tourette a voice that has been predominately silenced in both schools and the larger community. My only requirements were:

1. The teacher self-identified as an educator with Tourette syndrome;
2. They work or worked in a K-12 public school district; and
3. Their participation was voluntary.

There were no age, race, or ethnic requirements.

Data Collection

I applied for approval for my research through the university's Internal Review Board (IRB) process. After receiving approval, I went about conducting my research. I disseminated fliers about my research study, along with my contact information, through friends, colleagues, and advisors at the university, as well as my neurologist. I also used social networking by posting my flier on the Tourette Syndrome Association Facebook page. After selecting my participants, I held a telephone conversation with them to set up our first meeting time and location. This initial contact with them, even by phone, helped to build rapport between the interviewer and interviewees that continued the duration of the relationship, which lasted approximately two to three weeks. I asked each participant for some basic contact information, which I kept secure in my home office in a locked filing cabinet. I also took this opportunity to explain the study and its purpose. I introduced the informed consent form and explained what it covers; I explained that he or she will be provided with a consent form to sign and return to me, as well as one to keep, at our first meeting time.

With four participants, I conducted three interviews, spaced out between three days to one week for each interview. Therefore, the entire interview process took two to three weeks to complete (Seidman, 2006). Due to time constraints, three participants chose to conduct one longer interview. The time and location of each meeting was one that was convenient for the participant. Each of the three interviews lasted approximately 20-65 minutes. This time commitment allowed the relationship between the researcher and the interviewee to build in a positive manner. The interviewee knew that the researcher was truly interested in hearing what he or she had to say. The researcher demonstrated this interest by spending a significant amount of time with participants at each meeting.

Many interviewees felt respected and valued because they were asked to talk about their experiences and what the experiences meant to them. Many interviewees had never been asked to talk about their particular experiences before. This, in itself, was a way of creating a mutual respect between the researcher and participant. I continued my data collection via interviews until I reached saturation of information. Merriam (2009) summarizes what this means by explaining that you continue collecting data until the emerging findings feel saturated, meaning eventually, you hear the same things over and over again and no new information arises from collecting more data.

It was believed that participants may feel some emotional stress due to reflecting on and talking about past experiences. This can occur when one relives unpleasant past experiences by talking about them in the interview. If they needed help in dealing with the stress produced by re-experiencing past events, I referred them to the University's Family and School Counseling Center.

I digitally recorded each interview using a digital audio recorder. I transcribed each of the interviews myself in my home office. I kept the recordings saved in a password protected file on my personal computer; I will delete the audio recordings off my digital recorder after my manuscript is completed. All printed transcriptions, along with any contact information, were stored securely in a locked filing cabinet in my home office. During transcription, I removed all identifiable information, including names of people and school districts. My participants had the option of choosing their own pseudonyms for my study. Finally, as a way of increasing trustworthiness of data, I provided each participant with a transcription of all three interviews for feedback on the accuracy of the data; this process is called member checking.

Data Analysis

Data analysis began during transcription. To start the analysis of my data, I transcribed all the interviews myself. As I transcribed and read through the transcripts of my interviews, I kept a record of related themes or concepts, as well as my own thoughts and reflections, in a notebook. After I transcribed each of my interviews, I played the audio recording back while I reread them to double check for accuracy. After I ensured accuracy, I reread the transcripts a second time, this time circling common words or themes that recurred throughout the interviews. I also made notes in the margins of the transcripts. After I identified some common themes in the transcripts, I wrote each word or phrase on a small sticky note. From there, I took a large sheet of poster board, and grouped related sticky notes in clusters on the poster board.

This process gave me a plan with which I was able to picture the chapters on data analysis taking form. I had four groups which became the major concepts of my findings. The related sticky notes in each cluster became categories within each major concept. My four concepts dealt with how Tourette syndrome affected the participants' relationships with their administrators, colleagues, students and their parents, as well how Tourette syndrome shaped their own identity. After identifying my major concepts and categories, I went back and open and axial coded all my transcripts. As described by Merriam (2009), "Coding is nothing more than assigning some sort of shorthand designation to various aspects of your data so that you can easily retrieve specific pieces of data" (p. 173).

When I finished identifying my major concepts and emergent categories and open and axial coded all my transcripts, I created a character profile for each participant. As Seidman (2006) encouraged, I wrote the profiles in the words of the participant. I created the character profiles by reading each transcript and bracketing the passages of interest. Like Seidman (2006) discussed, this reduced the original transcript to between one third and one half the length of the original three-interview transcript. The character profiles represented a truncated version of the original transcript, narrating the participants lived experiences. After I completed the character profiles for each participant, I sent each person a copy of his or her profile. I asked participants to read them and let me know of any errors or issues I needed to clarify. I gave a copy of the respective transcript and character profile to each participant to ensure reliability, validity, and member-checking. This means of triangulation of data helped to ensure internal validity. Merriam (2009) describes triangulation as using multiple sources of data to compare and cross-check information, or to receive follow-up from interviews with the same person.

After identifying concepts and categories and creating character profiles, I laid out the framework for my research findings chapters. I drafted the interpretations and findings chapters after completing the exercise with the poster board and sticky notes. My analysis and findings are explored in depth in Chapters Four, Five, Six and Seven.

CHAPTER FOUR

PARTICIPANTS' JOURNEYS

Purpose

This chapter begins with a synopsis of each participant's personal and professional experiences. This chapter specifically focuses on: first memories of tics, when participants were diagnosed, how they feel about discussing Tourette syndrome with family members and friends, and how they view their role as an educator. The answers to these questions are important to establish a foundation to understand the lives of educators with Tourette syndrome. However, we cannot generalize that these experiences are the same for all educators with Tourette syndrome.

Participants' Journeys

Laura's Journey.

Laura is a 21 year old woman with Tourette syndrome. She has a master's degree and has been a teacher for one year. Last year, she taught 5th grade, but next year, she will teach 8th grade math. Laura first remembers having tics at about age six:

> It started out as vocal tics. I would clear my throat all the time, and I didn't know why, and I couldn't stop. I actually used to get, not really punished for it, but my mom would be like, "Why are you doing that? Stop doing that." But I could never stop. So I got really embarrassed about it. And I also had really bad obsessions: counting things and rituals and having to do things in certain order. And then

my parents just kind of told me, "Well, it's normal. You're fine," until I was in high school. When I was in high school, I really started noticing the motor tics. Mostly with my eyes. I blink a lot; I also do some shoulder shrugging and some neck twisting. Every once in a while, my head will completely go back. They kind of come and go. I have different tics at different times. But I was in the hospital when I was 17, my doctors finally diagnosed me with OCD. They were like, "You have really bad OCD. How was this never diagnosed?" Well, it turned out, both my parents have it, so they just thought it was totally normal. So I was diagnosed with OCD when I was 17. And then, the tics got worse and worse and worse. When I was in college, I actually went through a period of time where I wouldn't even leave my house because they were so embarrassing. They were constant. I had no breaks between any of them, so I would sit there completely twitching, and when I would go to class, people would stare at me. I was really embarrassed about it. When I was 19, I ended up in rehab for anorexia, which I had been struggling with at that point for about six or seven years. While I was in rehab, my psychiatrist kept telling me, "You have Tourette's." And I kept telling her, "No I don't. You are crazy. You are making this up." She kept slipping info sheets in my cubby, and I would just throw them away. And any time she brought it up, I would get really mad at her. I would say, "No, Tourette's is for crazy people. I am not crazy." And then finally, she convinced me to start going on some Tourette's meds. I did and saw what a difference it made. So since then, I've come to accept it. My medication controls it pretty well. I still have tics. They're not severe most of the time. They do get severe at times. When I'm tired, when

I'm anxious or stressed, overwhelmed. That's when
they come out really bad. (Laura 21 – 51)

It is not so easy for Laura to discuss Tourette syndrome with
everyone. In fact, it is with her own family that she finds it
hardest. When asked if she felt comfortable discussing her
Tourette's with family members, Laura responded:

Not at all. My mom doesn't, she won't admit that I
actually have it. She's very reluctant to. When I had
surgery just a couple of weeks ago, as I was waking
up from the anesthesia, I started having really bad
seizures. I vaguely remember this conversation, and
the neurologist came in, and I overheard them
talking about Tourette's. And my mom said, "Well,
she's got a Tourette's diagnosis, but I'm not really
comfortable with that, and I don't really think it's
true." Then when I woke up, she's like, "Guess
what? You don't have Tourette's." And I was like,
"The guy saw me unconscious, and you're taking
his opinion over someone I lived with, a
psychiatrist that I worked with for two months
intensively." So, I feel like she's ashamed of it. But
I have four cousins with Tourette's. I'm not
uncomfortable talking about it with some of my
cousins, but my parents, for sure, I don't like it.
(Laura 150 – 159)

Laura explained that her mom will yell at her all the time for
cracking her knuckles and joints, a tic because of her
Tourette's. She told me that she has to tell her mother, "I have
to. You don't get it." It can get complicated because popping
your knuckles is a habit for many people, but a tic is not just a
habit.

Just as her mother doesn't always understand her, we can be
misjudged by the community as well. Although Laura has

never experienced any discrimination at her workplace, she has been discriminated against in the community. She explained:

> Yeah, definitely other places. One place that really sticks out in my head, and it's kind of silly: I was getting my nails done for my sister's wedding. And I started ticcing really badly, and the guy, the manicurist, he just started laughing at me. He just didn't understand, and I tried to tell him, "It's Tourette's." But he didn't speak very good English, and so he just kept laughing at me. And I started crying. I was like, "This is ridiculous." How do you explain that to someone who doesn't speak English? It was embarrassing because all the other bridesmaids were there, and he was making fun of me in front of all of them. My parents call me Blinky. My dad will come up and be like, "Hey Blinky," and start winking at me and I'm like, "That's not funny. Do not do that." (Laura 242 - 249)

At times, the anxiety she experiences over the possibility of being discriminated against is so great, it locks up the doors around her:

> Well, sometimes when my tics are really bad, I find myself not wanting to leave my house. And so definitely, my social life is affected that way. I don't like to go to events with a lot of people because they get really bad, and inevitably, someone's going to start staring. In college, sometimes I felt like I couldn't go to class because they were really bad. I try not to let it affect me, but it's frustrating when I go to the grocery store or Target or something and they start happening, and people just kind of give you that look like, "What is wrong with you?" (Laura 230 – 235)

Although Laura avoided going to certain places because of having Tourette syndrome, there is always a place or two people feel most comfortable to tic. Laura, like myself, feels most comfortable to tic when she is alone at home. At home, no one is there to judge you or look at you strangely. However, if Laura has to tic around others, she feels most comfortable to tic when she is at church:

> Church, for sure. My church is really great, and I've never met anyone more accepting. So if I have to be around people and tic, those are the people I want to be around. (Laura 146 – 147)

Even though Laura is not comfortable discussing Tourette syndrome with her immediate family, she is totally comfortable discussing Tourette's with friends. That does not bother her at all.

Laura wanted to become an educator because school was a safe place for her:

> School was a safe haven for me when I was younger. I came from a rough family. I love my family very much, but we had some issues. And school was safe. I knew that I wasn't going to get hurt at school. I knew that I was good at school. I loved my teachers. I loved being around my friends. And I really, as an adult, I still love learning. I consider myself a lifelong learner. And really, I want to give kids that good start. I want them, in those early years, to learn to love school, and to learn to love to learn. Because if that happens, it will carry on throughout their adulthood. (Laura 75 – 81)

Laura's teaching style is fairly traditional. She bases her classroom on respect:

My kids know that it's unacceptable to shout out and to wear hats in the building and to wear their hoods up or say mean things about their classmates. Respect is really the basis of our classroom. Academically, I do like to do activities where the kids make their own meaning and really explore the content. I like to interact with them a lot. I'm pretty relaxed with the kids. They actually laugh at me because I sing and dance in front of them. I'm like, "Whatever." But we have a lot of fun. My class is fun. (Laura 193 – 198)

Respect is a key factor in education, and it is key to people with Tourette syndrome as well. We just want to be treated like everybody else. No better, no worse. Laura is using her role as an educator to instill respect in children. Hopefully, they will carry this with them their entire lives, as well as educate other people they interact with about the importance of respecting others.

Laura did not ask for any accommodations from her school district, nor did she need to make any for herself in order to be successful in the classroom. She did make accommodations for herself when working with her colleagues:

Not in my classroom. In staff meetings, I would generally sit in the back so that no one could see the tics. And they were fine with that. They knew why I did it. But in my classroom, no. (Laura 259 – 260)

In her years of elementary education, Laura does not remember being treated any differently by teachers or peers because of having Tourette:

My tics weren't bad in elementary and middle school. They were bad in very early elementary school, and then they kind of tapered off a little bit. I don't remember being treated any differently. I remember thinking I was really weird and not knowing what was going on, but I don't remember anyone noticing. (Laura 350 – 353)

Like many others with Tourette, she was teased and made fun of in high school:

High school is when they got a little worse. People used to mock my movements. They'd do it, or be like, "Hey, why are you winking at me?" Just silly stuff like that. And at that time I wasn't diagnosed with Tourette's, and so I would get really upset about it. "I don't know why I'm doing this. Why are you making fun of me?" Mostly they would just mock the movements I made. Teachers never did, obviously, but students. (Laura 355 – 359)

Laura credits some of her experiences in high school to influencing her wanting to become an educator:

In high school, I had a couple teachers who really became my protectors, I guess, and really helped me through. I was going through a really rough time in high school with Tourette's and the OCD and anxiety and just everything, and they were there for me every step of the way. And it made me want to be like that for some child who needed me to. (Laura 361 – 364)

Laura is a novice teacher who has her first year of teaching under her belt. Her voice is powerful in my research because it represents the beginning teacher in her early 20s, and shares with us the way an educator with Tourette syndrome handles the pressures and everyday demands of the teaching profession.

Michelle's Journey.

Michelle is a 40 year old woman with Tourette syndrome. She has been an educator for 15 years and works as a speech pathologist with children in kindergarten through 5th grade.

She has a master's degree. Michelle's tics are not very severe, but she is comfortable with Tourette because she has two children with it as well.

Michelle reflects on the beginning of her symptoms:

> I remember in grade school, I don't know what grade it was actually, but I remember being in grade school, and I'd always hidden my tics. I've never let other people see them. When I was in school, I would purposely drop something so that when I went to pick up my pencil from the floor next to my desk, I could tic. But I don't know how old I was. I actually have never officially been diagnosed. I figured out that I have Tourette's based on my daughter, when she was first diagnosed. So when we got the criteria for her is when I then talked to her neurologist and I said, "Gee, do I need to go to a doctor for it? I mean, that is clearly what I have." And because I don't need medication for it, I've never gone to a neurologist myself for it. Like I said, even around my kids, I don't tic a lot. They'll see me tic, but I tend to hide it just because that's how I've lived my life. As my kids get older, I show it more. I've had all sorts of tics. A lot of my tics are similar to my daughter's tics. The breathing tics, she has a breathing one. I did a lot of that, I tended to, because nobody knew what it was, my parents just told me to stop. Nobody knew what it was, so I just would try to stop. I would tic in the shower. I specifically remember doing that. I had a neck tic that I would do in the shower. And then I just, I think because I work so hard on hiding them, they were never as severe as my kids' tics. I mean they seemed easier for me to hide. I don't know if that is the case or not. Even when I dated my husband, and we got married and everything, I didn't know that that's what I had, so I would just hide the tics all the

time. Then again, it wasn't until my daughter was diagnosed nine years ago, that's when we went for her doctor appointment, and that's what I said to my husband, "Oh my gosh, that's what I have. Now it all makes sense." So since then, we've been able to look on both sides of our families actually and see that different people in both of our families, I think that whether or not they have Tourette's, they at least have chronic tic disorder. Well, it was nine years ago when my daughter, she actually started ticcing before that. She was about three whenever she started ticcing, but she wasn't diagnosed until she turned six. And it was when we went to the first doctor which, ironically enough, we went to the doctor because the kindergarten teacher said, "I think you should go to the doctor." And while I was working the one-year temporary position that I mentioned, I was working with an occupational therapist who is a very good friend of mine now, and her name is Amy, and she actually at lunch, just through conversation, said, "It sounds like you should have your kids see this wonderful doctor here," so that's where we got the name. Then we went to the pediatrician for her, and the pediatrician said, "I think you should see this doctor," and it was the same doctor. It was kind of funny how that worked out. So once she was diagnosed, and we had the criteria in our hands that we could read through, that's when I said, "Well, this makes sense. This is what I have." (Michelle 17 – 41)

Because Michelle was often told to stop ticcing, she, like many people with Tourette, feels most comfortable to tic when she is alone. Michelle prefers to tic in the car. Even though people can see her, there is a sense of isolation in being in a car by yourself:

In my car, which is kind of funny if you think about it because there's people everywhere. But I do, I think in my car. I think maybe because when I'm out somewhere, I work so hard on not ticcing, that then I get in my car, it's my own place. So I definitely tic more when I am in my car. At home I tic too, but I tic more if I'm alone in a room than I do if my family is in the room with me. (Michelle 186 – 190)

As a mother with two children with Tourette syndrome, Michelle is extremely comfortable in discussing Tourette with family members. It is a typical topic of conversation for her immediate family. She is fairly comfortable discussing Tourette with friends, but it is not as easy as with her family:

I guess my close friends, I would say equally as comfortable as my family. People, we have a tight group of friends that we all hang out, and they all know, it's just out there. I guess more casual acquaintances, definitely not as comfortable. (Michelle 196 – 198)

Although Michelle does not think her Tourette has affected her in the community much because she is so adept at hiding her tics, she has been affected in the community by being the mother of two children with Tourette syndrome:

My son, particularly, his tics are much louder. For example, there is a breathing tic that he used to do. He doesn't do it so much anymore, but we would be in church and people would hear him breathe and think, "The kid's having an asthma attack," for example. And he's not having an asthma attack, but they're looking at me like, "Why are you not helping your child?" And church is a place where you can't simply address it. We always joke that we must be fun to watch at Disney World because between me and my two kids, we're ticcing up Main Street USA. We must be comical. One time we were on the trip, my son was having his breathing tic, and we're standing in line for some ride, I can't remember what the ride was, he keeps doing his breathing tic, and of course, you know they're going to tic way more than they do at home, and he's doing this breathing tic, and I'm talking to my husband, I'm not really paying attention to the people around us. And my daughter saw this woman looking. She's looking at my son; she's looking at me; she's looking at my son; she looks at me. My daughter, who is very outspoken, nicely says, "Oh, it's just a tic, he can't help that. He's just fine. That's just what it is." So the woman of course was terribly embarrassed. She turned around like, "Oh my God," just totally embarrassed. But that's just us. We're just open about it, and if someone in the community does say something, any one of us is going to just put it out there. Not in a mean way. My kids know that everyone is not aware of it. We just try to educate as we go. (Michelle 265 – 281)

Michelle describes her own teaching style as open:

I'm pretty open with the kids. I let them run the, I mean I have my goals, but I let them drive where we're going to go. Most of the time, there is some sort of game involved in what we're doing. The game is typically not relevant to what the activity is. So they really feel like they're leading the activity because they get to choose that. And none of my kids are working on the same goal ever, almost ever. So if I have three kids, there are three different goals. But by just doing some sort of board game, it keeps them all involved. And then they get to all practice their oral skills. (Michelle 218 – 224)

She truly loves being an educator:

> Well it sounds so cliché, but I really love it. The
> kids that I work with, there's a real need for what I
> do. Working with the same kids over a long period
> of time, I get to see them come into the special
> education piece of it, and then many times I get to
> see them move out of it, if they don't need the
> therapy anymore. Sometimes they need more
> services, and that's okay too. But I really love it. I
> love what I do. I like kids; I like to watch them
> grow. I just really like it. (Michelle 371 – 375)

Although Michelle loves being an educator, her own school experiences did not influence her desire to become an educator. Michelle did not recall being treated any differently in elementary or high school by teachers or peers because of having Tourette. This was most likely because she was so good at masking her tics, something that only people with mild cases of Tourette are able to do:

> You know what; I didn't know that I had Tourette's,
> so my teachers didn't know. I don't remember, I
> ticced but I really ticced mostly by myself or I
> worked really hard to hide it, so I don't think that
> anyone really knew, to be honest. (Michelle 392 –
> 394)

Even in high school, Michelle was able to mask her tics:

> And I got better at hiding it as I got older. You get
> past those puberty years, and life is a little bit
> different. (Michelle 396 – 397)

Michelle's story offers a unique perspective of the life of an educator with Tourette syndrome. Michelle is in the middle part of her career, having been in education for 15 years. Not only is she an educator with Tourette syndrome, she is also the mother of two children with Tourette. Her experiences in both her professional life and in the community in general offer a great insight in understanding the lives of educators with Tourette syndrome.

Jason's Journey.

Jason is an elementary school teacher with his bachelor's degree. He has been a teacher for six years. He has taught special education for three years and sixth grade science for three years. Next year, he will teach a fifth grade classroom all subject matters.

Jason first remembers having tics around age eight or nine:

> I was not formally diagnosed, but when I was about 28 years old, I always kind of knew something was weird with me. As far as back as eight or nine years old, I always made humming noises or weird noises, I sniffed a lot, coughed a lot. My parents always thought it was allergies. That was probably when I was about 10 years old. And probably into my middle school and high school years is whenever I finally, to myself, thought something was different about me, as far as what I did and what my peers had done. But I never really looked into why I did it; I just figured maybe it was just habits because that's what my parents always thought too. Besides allergies, they thought it was habits. Habits I never outgrew, apparently. I ticced, I shake my head, my neck a lot, like body tics now more so than the vocal. I still cough a lot. But I didn't realize, really, that I did that; again, it's just something that I just did. I didn't realize it until my wife, we'd been married probably five or six years, and I was really good at hiding, holding in my tics when no one was looking. And I think being a teacher, for me, it's easier to hold them in. Like I

said, my wife never really realized it, I think she just again, thought it was part of me, and who I was. And then one day, I was sitting in the recliner, shaking my head and she asked, "Why are you doing that? I just now noticed that." And again we'd been married five or six years by that time. It took her a while to even notice that I did it. It kind of embarrassed me at the time, and I said, "You know, I don't know. I've always just kind of done that." And I think the head tics at that time were getting worse because I was looking for a job too. So, she talked me into going to the doctor, just a regular doctor. They told me to videotape myself and give them a family history, so I was just watching a football game, and I videotaped myself just watching the game, and took it into her. My grandma kind of had a tic disorder too. She shook her head a lot and coughed, and of course she's older, and they didn't really diagnose Tourette's back then. What I think now is she might have had a slight case of it like I have. But that's what the doctor said, "I think it is," and she referred me to a neurologist. I didn't go because I thought, "You know, I've lived with this my whole life. I don't need a doctor to tell me what I already know." I wasn't going to go on medicine because I've read a lot of books and watched a lot of videos over it, and everything I've ever read or heard about medicine is bad. And it puts you in a comatose state, and I don't want to go around like a zombie, so I just never did go to the neurologist to be formally diagnosed. But again, I don't need somebody to tell me what I already know. I remember back to probably 8 to 10 years old. I just remember my cousins kind of always teasing me about making noises and stuff. I just kind of blew it off back then. I didn't really know why I did it, but I did. (Jason 14 – 46)

Jason is more comfortable talking with people about Tourette now than when he was first diagnosed:

> When I first found out, in 2005, I was pretty secretive. I'd barely even told my in-laws or parents. (Jason 128 – 129)

When Jason was first diagnosed with Tourette syndrome, his mother did not want to believe it:

> My parents always kind of knew something was weird, but my mom has that old sense of, well, whenever I first said, "Well mom, I went to the doctor, and the doctor said, 'Yes, you definitely have Tourette's,'" she said, "But you're so smart." And I'm like, "Mom, that doesn't mean anything." I guess she thinks it's special ed like I was disabled or whatever. And she said, "But you don't cuss." Well that's not the main thing about it. It's a rare part of it, coprolalia. [Coprolalia is the exclamation of obscene words or socially inappropriate and derogatory remarks.] So I've been talking to her about it of course, but I was very leery about coming out and telling people that I had Tourette's. (Jason 129 – 135)

Although he is now comfortable talking with his parents about Tourette, he is not comfortable in discussing it with his brother or his in-laws:

> My mom and dad, I'm fine. My brother is still in denial, so I'm not really comfortable with him. He's still in denial; he's like, "Oh, whatever." I don't know. I think because he made fun of me for so many years, he's probably upset that he's done it, and he's ashamed of it or something. I don't know, but I'm not comfortable with him. But with my wife, I'm fine. My kids, I talk to my children about it, and I don't see any signs of them having it yet.

But mainly my mom and dad and my wife. My in-laws, not really. I don't feel comfortable with them either. (Jason 216 – 221)

He does feel fairly comfortable discussing Tourette with friends. As with many of us with Tourette, the more comfortable you are with a person, the easier it is to talk to them about sensitive subjects:

Once I get to know them, I'm fine. (Jason 223)

Jason describes his own teaching style as exploratory:

I'm more hands-on. I like kids to learn discovery wise. I don't like the direct, lecturing approach. Again, I taught science for three years, so that was pretty well the mode, the whole hands-on, do labs and activities, rather than book and vocab and things like that. I like the enrichment value. You know students are getting the topic, you give them more of a chance to delve deeper into the subject we're learning about, and then, of course, the kids who aren't up to speed, being able to work one-on-one with them while the other kids are working ahead. Now that I'm going to be teaching all the subjects, I'm going to try to keep that style going. Of course, I want to continue to keep science as a big focus because I think in elementary school, science is put on the back burner. It seems like reading and math are the main subjects, and science is on the back burner, but I'd like to be able to incorporate science with math and reading. (Jason 256 – 266)

While Jason has never asked for accommodations from his school district, he has made some for himself in order to be successful in the classroom:

No, I've never asked for any. The only thing I've probably ever done is maybe the arrangement of the room. It really doesn't have to do with the arrangement of the room, I guess, I just always leave room at the back like when the kids are facing the other direction so if I do need to get a tic out, if I'm particularly stressed, I can go back behind them when they're looking at the front of the room and get a tic out and then walk back around them. I do that kind of thing. (Jason 321 – 325)

Like many people with Tourette syndrome, Jason was mocked in high school by others. What was shocking in Jason's case is that he was mocked by one of his teachers:

Elementary, I was too young to really realize anything. I didn't notice it probably until high school, a physics teacher in high school, it's when I blinked a lot and cleared my throat a lot. I just remember the one thing, the only thing I really remember in high school was we were sitting there taking notes and the teacher was lecturing, and I was blinking and coughing, and he looked at me and he just started blinking and kind of mimicking me. And at that time, again, I had no idea, I just did that. I just thought that was what I did. And that's always stuck in my head. Why would a teacher do that? I don't know. Again I think it was just something different that the teacher had never encountered, and he just thought it was funny. I don't know. But that always stuck in my head. (Jason 361 – 369)

Jason believes this treatment in high school did affect his reasons for wanting to become an educator:

I would say probably yes, subconsciously it did. Just because I don't want students to have to go through that. Kids that have a learning disability or they might make different motions or whatever, they don't need to be mimicked because they're already dealing with that themselves. It definitely had an influence on me. (Jason 372 – 375)

Jason's story is strong in my research because it gives voice to an educator in the early stages of his career and how he handles being an educator with Tourette syndrome. Like all of my participants, he offers a unique perspective of what his journey has been like. Jason is another strong example of how people with Tourette syndrome can persevere beyond the disability and become a successfully working professional.

Tracey's Journey.

Tracey is 30 years old. She has been teaching for four years. She has taught fifth grade and now teaches third grade, all subjects. Tracey has her master's degree. She was diagnosed with Tourette syndrome when she was six years old. She remembers that her childhood was a rough one, as it was hard for her to make friends because of having Tourette syndrome:

I remember that it was really hard for me to make friends because I was always ticcing, making noises. I remember when I was first diagnosed, my parents actually thought I was having a seizure. I developed this head tic where I was bending my head back. They actually called the hospital, and I remember being rushed to the hospital and admitted into the hospital for a week because they didn't know what was going on. They thought it was the middle child syndrome, and they said I was doing it for attention. I remember my mom finally taking me to a hospital in a bigger city where the doctor within a half an hour had diagnosed me with Tourette's syndrome. It was very hard growing up with the disorganization skills, the ticcing, the OCD, because I have OCD with it. I remember locking, before I'd go to bed at night, I'd have to lock all the dollhouses. And I would have to even as an adult. I finally went back on medication because my husband woke up one morning at 2:00, and I'm searching my house. And we didn't know what I was searching for, I was just searching my house for stuff. I had to make sure things were in order before I went to bed. In college, my professors always thought I was disagreeing with them because I was shaking my head and the vocal noises that I made. I remember not having a lot of friends because I was kind of known as a freak. Because you did different motions that you weren't sure about. I remember going to school every day and getting picked on and not having friends and coming home and just fighting with my parents. I would have a bad day, and I would just let it out. It was like as soon as I got home, I felt a weight lifted off me, almost like I had spent all day enduring this negativity. And then I came home and everything, you just felt comfortable. But on the same token, my parents would say one thing to me, and I would just unleash. I remember the different medications. One medication I was on, Prozac, I can remember throwing dining room furniture. I would get mad at my mom, and I would tip over chairs. And it was hard. I think it was harder for my brother and sister because my father used to say, I would hear him talking to my mom and saying, "She's a handicapped child, and we have to be careful with her." And my brother and sister didn't understand it. I remember my mom calling my grandmother, my dad's mother, and she would call her on the phone and say, "You have to come take her. I can't deal with her anymore." Because it was aggression. It was that pent up anger from what you are going through every day. (Tracey 17 – 31, 33 – 46)

Tracey's teaching style is affected by her Tourette syndrome and associated disorders. Although she likes team teaching, she prefers working and planning alone in her room. She knows that because of her obsessive compulsive disorder, she tends to try to take on too much, as well as get distracted from what she is working on:

> I like to do things on my own, if that makes any sense. I like team teaching. I like collaborating with my colleagues, but I prefer to be by myself in the classroom doing things. In fact, it's funny because the kids, I've learned to stop myself and designate jobs to them because I feel like I can do everything on my own. But I also know I get very distracted, like sometimes I start ticcing, and that takes away from my planning time because I'm so busy doing that and my mind wanders. I'm multitasking, but it's weird because my mind carries away. I start organizing books, and then I see something across the room, and the next thing I know I'm across the room for 20 minutes doing stuff with computers and things like that, and then I'm like, "Oh shoot, I forgot the original thing I meant to go back to." (Tracey 177 – 185)

A typical work day for Tracey involves taking her Tourette syndrome, along with some of the associated disorders, into account:

> I get up. I usually walk around the house a little bit. I check, just to make sure there are no lights on, that the stove wasn't on during the night, little OCD things. I get ready. I kind of putter around the house. I get to school. I try to leave, I have to try to leave by 7:15 because before I leave, it's like the

typical routine where I have to check and make sure the stove is off, check to make sure all the lights are off, check to make sure the doors are closed, all that good stuff. And then, I don't know, I get to work at 7:30. I need a few minutes to unwind. Then I get into my day at school. (Tracey 169 – 175)

Although Tracey has not asked for accommodations at work, she has made some for herself in order to be successful:

I haven't asked for accommodations, but in terms of myself, I do know that my hardest thing is focusing with time. I know that I get distracted, I know that, even before I leave the classroom, I feel like I have to have things on my desk in a certain way. Before I leave, my husband laughs, at the end of the day, if he picks me up from work or something and I say, "I'll be down at 3:45," it's probably going to be closer to 4:00 or 4:30 because by the time I check to make sure my desk is cleaned off and that the lights are all off and that the door is locked, I check the computers 50 different times, I know that it's going to take me a while to get to my destination. So I kind of make accommodations with myself in knowing that I need to start leaving class a few minutes earlier and knowing that I need to focus on one task at hand too because otherwise I would begin six and seven tasks and never complete one of them. But I started six or seven of them. (Tracey 268 – 277)

Tracey wanted to become a teacher because of the good teachers she had growing up. She also wanted to be the kind of teacher who supported kids and was there for everyone:

I had some really good teachers growing up. I went to Catholic school for a couple of years. As I got older, I just really cherished what they did for me.

They kind of took me under their wing and helped me out. And I decided that I wanted, there were other kids that didn't have this great of teachers, and I wanted to be the kind of teacher that understood every disability and could provide a safe environment that my teachers had provided for me. (Tracey 51 – 55)

She feels like being a teacher is a part of her now. She relates to the adage, "Once a teacher, always a teacher":

The emotional connections between my life and work, teaching for me has really, it's become my life. I think any teacher will tell you, you're always a teacher no matter where you are. My husband always laughs because he'll sometimes say I'm teacher talking him. You can't really get that out of your system. So it's very emotional. It's emotional. Sometimes you have very stressful days. And I come home, and I'm ticcing uncontrollably. If something happens to me, like when that parent got upset with me for having the Tourette's, and then I come home, I feel like teaching is an emotional roller coaster with you. But, I don't know it's always, it's happy with me. I love doing my job. And I love coming home. So I feel like that's just a part of me. (Tracey 389 – 396)

Similar to many people with Tourette syndrome, Tracey feels most comfortable to tic at home. When you are by yourself or around people who know and understand you best, you can relax and feel free to tic without being judged by others. Tracey considers her own house, her parents' house, and her in-laws' house all home. These are the places she feels the most comfortable to tic because she feels like she is in her safest environment.

As she feels so comfortable ticcing at home, she also feels extremely comfortable talking with family members about Tourette syndrome:

> Very comfortable. Just growing up, I think my parents, even going through that whole diagnosis, we went through a lot to get the diagnosis, so I think my family just understands what I was going through. And they're very welcoming with it. (Tracey 141 – 143)

Likewise, she is also very comfortable talking with friends about Tourette:

> Very comfortable. My friends are very understanding. They're very nonjudgmental. They understand. So I feel like I'm very comfortable discussing it with them. (Tracey 145 – 146)

However, she has not always felt open to discussing Tourette with friends. She was not comfortable talking about it with friends in high school:

> No, not until I got older. As you get older you find more and more, like when I joined the Tourette's organization, when I rejoined when I was in college, that's when I started getting more comfortable with it. But back in high school, you tried to hide it. You didn't want anyone to know that you are different. But I find for myself that as I get older, I don't really have a problem with it. (Tracey 148 – 152)

Tracey has felt the effects of discrimination and lack of understanding about Tourette syndrome in the community:

> As I get older, I find it's not as bad, but I do know that during the movies, when I have to make the vocal tics, people think you're shushing them. I also

find out in the community, when I was in college and I would shake my head, professors thought that I was disagreeing with them. And I think even when you're talking to someone and you do that, that their first reaction is, she doesn't agree with what I'm saying. I don't know, I feel like you can blend in more now. When I was younger, restaurants were harder, movies were harder. You stood out like a sore thumb. But maybe it's because there's so many more disabilities coming to light now days, that I don't feel it's as bad as it used to be. Although like I said, you're still self-conscious. You're in a crowd of people or you're in the class or you're giving a presentation, you're like, "Oh my goodness, here I am shaking my head and making these noises." (Tracey 247 – 256)

Opposed to facing discrimination in the community, Tracey has worked to provide a safe harbor for children with Tourette syndrome. She has worked as a counselor for a summer camp devoted to children with Tourette. She recalls that it is a very accepting and comforting place for a child with Tourette to spend time each summer:

Every year, they have a camp where they call it Ticapalooza. It's a weekend camp. The kids get there Friday at maybe 4:00 and goes till Sunday afternoon. But it's all kids with Tourette's syndrome. And it's really enjoyable. I did it a couple years in a row, and I was a counselor. It is phenomenal. You get together with kids of all ages up to 18 that have Tourette's, and then some of the adults end up being counselors. It's funny to see everybody with Tourette's there. That whole camp, everyone has Tourette's. And they have relay races and campfires and there is a guy who does a drumming circle. I remember the first year I went to it, and I was like, "Wow." They have different counseling sessions, and they have different seminars and guest speakers. But piggybacking off of what you said, it's nice to sit around and talk to other people with Tourette's, for kids to talk to other kids. And for you to look at the kids and say, "Oh my goodness, I remember doing that when I was younger. I remember how they're feeling." And even talking to the younger adults, and saying the same thing, like, "Oh my goodness, I didn't know anybody else felt the same way I did or went through and understood what I'm going through." It's a phenomenal camp. (Tracey 308 – 322)

Elementary school was very difficult for Tracey, as she had trouble making friends because of her Tourette syndrome:

It was not a happy time for me. I went to a Catholic school until I was in third grade. And that was fine because it was a private school, and everyone got along. My teachers were always understanding. But as I had, I don't know, my teachers have not been too bad. My mom has been my biggest advocate, in that sense, always having meetings with teachers and helping them understand. In terms of peers, it was just not a good time. I didn't have a lot of friends. I was made fun of a lot. I was very isolated. I remember my sister and my brother were always out having fun, and I was a child that was in my room reading or crying. And you look back on that, when I got into high school, it kind of got a little bit better, but for most of my years, you feel just isolated from everybody else. You feel different. I feel as a society, we're getting better. Children are becoming more understanding that 15, 20 years ago, people didn't know a lot about Tourette's. Kids can be very, very cruel. And even teachers. I think they expect a lot from you, and they don't like you disrupting their class. They don't always understand the things that you do. (Tracey 411 – 423)

I very much relate to Tracey's feelings of isolation. Starting around fourth grade, I would always go into my bedroom after school and shut the door. I would always say I was doing homework or reading a book; really what I was doing was isolating myself so I could tic in private without anyone watching me. I very much isolated myself this way. Even when I was in college and lived in an apartment with my sister, I would shut the door when I was in my room.

High school, although a little bit better for Tracey, was still tough:

> Like I said, in high school, it got a little bit better. I had a little group of friends, and I really enjoyed myself. Still, a lot of kids didn't understand. You really felt like a freak. I spent all day suppressing the tics and came home and let them out. It just was a very, very hard time. Kids don't understand. And the teachers, you know I think in high school they got better because my mom worked at the school. But I know my sister and brother had a lot of teachers, and my mom would fight not to have me in those classes because she knew they just wouldn't understand. (Tracey 425 – 430)

Tracey does believe that this treatment in school had an influence on her wanting to become a teacher:

> It did because I really felt like I could make a huge difference. I felt like I could be, in elementary school I had a lot of great teachers, and I wanted to be that type of teacher. And I wanted to be the type of teacher that kids, I wanted kids to want to come to my classroom. I didn't want them to feel like they didn't want to come to class, they were scared to come to class, not because of me, because of other

kids. And I really felt like I give an atmosphere that was very supportive, where they would want to learn, and they would want to come to class, and they could confide in me, and school would be fun for them. I mean, maybe not all the time with learning. But I just, I wanted to be an important role model for them. And I really felt like I had a few teachers that did that, and I had a few that didn't. But I wanted to be that perfect teacher to really help out the kids. (Tracey 432 – 441)

Tracey's story provides a lens to examine the life of a young teacher with Tourette syndrome. She has reflected on her own schooling and how this makes her want to be a better teacher for children who need a positive role model in their lives. Although not all of Tracey's experiences in teaching have been positive, she feels supported and backed by family members and her administrators at all times. She is a true example of someone who is successful in life, despite any obstacles she has had to overcome.

Mike's Journey.

Mike is 37 years old. He has been an educator for 15 years. He has taught second and third grades, all subjects. Mike has his master's degree and his specialist degree. He remembers a great deal about the start of his tics:

I first recognized my tics in fourth grade. I started making vocal tics. When I first started doing it, not many people knew what was going on. There wasn't much education about Tourette's. My mom was trying to figure out what was going on, where my dad thought I could stop it. That I could control it. Then I was soon after diagnosed. And then we were able to educate people about Tourette's. When I was in school, I had difficult times. My teachers didn't understand what was going on. They didn't want to believe us. They thought that they had their own remedies to fix the problem. They often put me in the corner to learn. They kicked me out of class. They put me in in-school suspension. They pretty much didn't believe me. They saw me as the problem child. They wanted to put the problem child away. I tried to be as normal as anybody else. I wanted to be treated as anybody else. I just had to figure it out on my own. I had a supportive family to a degree, but at the same time, they were trying to figure out why. I remember in middle school, teachers kicking me out of class; I remember I didn't have any friends; I remember eating lunch alone. I remember they didn't know what to do with me. I think they thought I was a good kid, that I just had this problem, but it was just a big problem when you looked at academics. And then in middle school, we had the opportunity to start educating people about Tourette's. And what we realized was that as soon as we started educating people, they were actually more compassionate than you thought. We started with the kids. And as soon as the students knew what was going on, typically the teachers followed suit. And life started to get a little better for me. When I got to high school, I started to have a little more of a social life. My self-esteem went up, my academic grades went up because I didn't have to worry about getting kicked out of class or not having any friends or other kids picking on me. In middle school, I was definitely bullied a lot. But once I got to high school, people started respecting me a little bit more. They knew what it was, and they just left you alone. So I wasn't picked on anymore. So I actually had a pretty good high school experience. I joined the youth group; I joined other extracurricular activities at school. I took on leadership roles. I started doing things. (Mike 20 – 44)

Mike remembers his reason for wanting to become an educator:

As I got older, I knew I needed to figure out what I wanted to do with my life, and I knew that I wanted to be a teacher. I wanted to be that educator that was focused on the kids' strengths, not their weaknesses. I knew what it was like for a teacher not to believe in me, and I knew that it shouldn't be that way. My goal was that I wanted to be that teacher that I never had. I decided to go to college. I went to college for four years. After I got on the college campus, I educated people about Tourette's. Again, those people, for the most part, they embraced me. Some of them didn't want to have anything to do with me; they just left me alone. I didn't have any problems. For four years, I studied hard. I had a great social life. I had really good experiences. I knew I was going to become a teacher. I graduated in four years, graduated with honors. I decided to take on the world, and go out and be that teacher that I knew I could be, and follow my dream. (Mike 45 – 54)

Mike describes his own teaching style as always looking at the bigger picture:

I definitely tried to always make that connection to the real world. I allowed my students to understand that it's not just about the textbook. They were learning for a much bigger picture. And there are going to be challenges, but we're going to get through them. I taught them to learn that you're going to have to be able to make mistakes. When I was going through education, every time I made a mistake, I had someone reminding me that I messed up. And that's not how it should be. Students should be able to learn, and students should be able to go through trial and error, and mess up. Then figure things out. Figure how they're going to do it better next year. And that's what I try to do. I always try to give my students a choice in things that we do. I try to make their voice heard. I let them help create the rules of the classroom to maybe doing a project creatively, how I might grade them. I tried to show that the voice of the students is a powerful thing. You need to have the students buy into what you're doing. It makes the challenges of the classroom, pretty much, disappear. (Mike 201 – 212)

A typical workday for Mike was fast paced:

I wake up about 5:15 or 5:30. Get dressed. Take care of stuff around the house. Take care of all the extracurricular stuff. Do what I've got to do, and then get to work. I always got to work early. I was one of those people that, if I'm not ready, how are the kids going to be ready? I was usually at school at least 20 minutes, a half-hour before the kids got there. Did my thing at school. Taught, taught, taught. Always on the go. Run, run, run. Do what I did. And when school was over, I was one of those people that, I never brought work home. I always left it there. Too many distractions at home. So I would often stay until 5:00, maybe 5:30. Get everything done, graded their papers. Planning lessons, collaborating with my cohort. Putting all the materials together, decorating the room, tutoring, whatever it was. Then I get home, eat dinner. I also did a lot of extracurricular things like playing sports or being involved in organizations, tutoring, giving back in some way. Later in my life, it was writing a book. Later in life, it was being married and being with my family. Always get a little TV time in, watch the sports. Then I'd eventually go to bed. I usually don't jump into bed until least 11. I've done that most of my life. (Mike 182 – 194)

Mike is an extremely dedicated educator. He talks about the intellectual and emotional connections between his life and work being one of passion:

I just have a passion for whatever I do. I try to give 100 percent. Do what's best for whatever the cause is. And I love making a difference. I love educating. I tried to bring that passion to the classroom every single day. I tried to show my students that they need to have a positive attitude, life isn't going to be easy. It's okay to have a negative attitude, but at some point you've got to make that switch and get back to having a positive attitude. I think it's about perseverance. Never giving up, never making excuses. Yeah you can, but you shouldn't. People don't like other people just walking around making excuses for their life all day. Everyone has problems. You might not necessarily see another person's problems. It could be the loss of a job or a death in the family, and it could be something like a learning disability that you just don't see. Mine is very visible and you see it, but I don't make excuses, so hopefully you won't either. (Mike 297 – 306)

Most people with Tourette syndrome have a place where they feel most comfortable to tic. Unlike many other of my participants who felt most comfortable to tic at home or when they are alone, Mike felt most comfortable to tic in his classroom:

The classroom. You know, that's my home, so let me do my thing. I don't suppress my tics. I do what I do. And whatever happens, happens. I wouldn't say there's a place I like doing my tics more. Obviously there's places I don't like doing them as much. If you go to movie theaters or restaurants, there's definitely more uncomfortable places the more quiet it gets, but in regards to a place I like doing it more, there really isn't a place, but in a way, it's kind of like my classroom was my home. I was there from seven in the morning to 5:30, 6:00 at night. If I was not going to be comfortable in my own classroom, I would never be an effective teacher. (Mike 148 – 154)

Mike is fairly comfortable discussing Tourette syndrome with his family, but he does not always enjoy it. In fact, at times he gets tired of discussing it with family:

I would say in the big picture, if I take a step back, I don't necessarily like talking about it. I don't like talking about it from a point of view that, I don't see it as a problem. People sit around and talk about their problems. There is nothing I hate more in life than to sit around and talk about your problems. I don't like going to therapists and counselors and sitting around talking about it. I don't care what it is. I don't care what the problem is. I'm not that kind of person. And I'm not saying I'm better than anybody else; some people, they need that. But for me, I didn't need to sit around and talk about it. This is just who I was. Sometimes my father would say, "Your noises are louder now." Well, thanks, thanks Dad. That's a great observation. You're very perceptive. I don't need to sit here and talk about that. I don't want to talk about it; it happens, and let's move on. If I want to talk about it, I'll talk about it. But with that being said, with my mom I

was a lot more open than with my dad. My dad
always wanted to fix it. My mom just wanted to
figure it out. And know how to move forward. So
we did talk about it. It's not like, "Oh, taboo, we
can't talk about Tourette's." It's not that at all. It's
more like, talk about it in a positive way. "Oh, look
how Mike's helping out the kids. And how he's
lived with Tourette's. Or look how he's written this
book." You know, the positive aspects. It's not
sitting around and talking about the negatives.
(Mike 156 – 171)

Although Mike faced discrimination in the community
while growing up, it hasn't been a problem lately:

It wasn't a negative thing at all. I think it's just
really a part of who I have been. I've always taken
on the extracurricular things and try to help other
people in the community. I've helped people
embrace it with me. And if I wanted to do
something to help others, they were willing to help
out. They knew it was my passion to help others. I
just never looked at it as a visible thing. I'm not
saying that life was always easy and that it wasn't
sometimes an issue. But what I do know is that
attitude is everything. Other people would see that
it wasn't a problem for me, and they realized that it
didn't need to be a problem for them. (Mike 233 –
239)

Mike does remember facing continual discrimination in
elementary and middle school because of having Tourette
syndrome. He vividly remembers elementary and middle
school:

Horrible. I had no friends. I was bullied. I
remember eating lunch in the cafeteria and all the
kids would pick on me, and when I looked up, there

wasn't one teacher that came to save me. They saw it. They turned their heads. They turned a blind eye to it. They didn't want to deal with it. Here I was, I knew that they saw what was going on, but no one wanted to save me. I just kind of took it like a man. And I did the best I could. You got to do what you got to do. You've got to figure it out. (Mike 314 – 319)

Fortunately for Mike, things did get a little easier in high school:

High school definitely got better. I've learned that education is a powerful tool. And that's why I decided I wanted to devote my life to it, and to be an educator. I realized that I should take advantage of every single opportunity and to be open and honest and to educate people about Tourette's syndrome. I knew the more people that I could educate, the better it would be for my life. As I got older, I kept saying I'm going to keep doing this because not only is it good for me, but hopefully it will be better for generations to come. We really have come a long way. In the 80s, there was not a lot of education about Tourette's and now there's tons. I think that's important. There are so many people that are my age or even older that did a lot of legwork, and we had to go through a lot of things that people now don't have to go through. But that's okay. That's part of the burden that's been put on our shoulders to try to make the world a better place. We're not here for sympathy. We're here to say that we went through it, and if we can make the lives of other kids a little easier than it was for us, then we're doing a good thing. (Mike 321 – 333)

Because of how he was treated in school, Mike wanted to be a teacher in order to become the teacher he never had. He wanted to be a positive role model in children's lives and support all children in his classroom. Mike's story is a representation of an educator with Tourette syndrome midway through his teaching career. Mike can show us all how people with disabilities, in this case Tourette syndrome, can persevere and do remarkable things in life. Mike makes a difference in countless lives because he clearly remembers the lack of support he received in school.

Stacy's Journey.

Stacy is a 30 year old teacher with her master's degree. She has taught music education to kindergarten through 6th grade for five years. She first remembers having symptoms of Tourette syndrome around age five:

> I think I first had tics when I was five. I think I got pretty bad when I was around seven. I think I was maybe diagnosed when I was seven or nine or something, sometime around there. My family was really, they never told me to stop or anything. They were pretty supportive. But I did have to go, when I was maybe in third grade, I had to go for a lot of testing and they poked me a lot for allergies, and I was actually seen by Dr. Atkins in New York City. He put me on a sugar-free diet, which I think helped because I also had a lot of tantrums and issues like that. I think that actually helped me, but I don't know if it was just all the attention also. I was able to suppress my tics. It was a lot of attention because I went to the doctor all the time. But I think that made me actually feel better. Mostly, people didn't make a big deal about it for me. I remember in third grade my teacher had asked me if I wanted to tell everyone or if I wanted her to do it, and I told her to do it when I wasn't there. So I don't know how it went over, but nobody ever said anything to me. Nobody ever brought it up in any real negative

ways. My grandmother would bribe me to stop doing things. Like I used to suck on my lip, and I used to bite my nails, so she used to bribe me with diamonds to stop. So it worked because I was able to stop sucking on my lip and start sucking on my tongue which no one ever noticed, and she gave me a diamond ring. But I really didn't stop, I just kind of transferred it. I've done a lot of transferring tics in order to not get attention. Childhood, I mean; as I got older, it got less noticeable. (Stacy 14 – 32)

She remembers being diagnosed:

I think I was seven. My teacher started noticing when I was five. I didn't even know I was doing anything. I don't think anyone ever really brought it to my attention. So being diagnosed, I don't remember being diagnosed. I was so young. I'm sure my parents took it pretty hard. I know my grandparents were blaming my mom because they didn't understand. They would say it was her fault for the way she was raising me. I'm not sure they really knew what it was. I did have to go to a lot of doctors, I remember that. And they were trying to send me to the best doctors in New York City. They don't talk about it now. (Stacy 57 – 63)

Stacy has a mild case of Tourette and does not find it difficult to suppress her tics at work:

Not necessarily. Sometimes it's a little weird, but I've gotten very good at playing it off as other things and being a little quirky. I don't think most people know. I don't tell most people. (Stacy 73 – 74)

Like several other participants in this study, Stacy is most comfortable ticcing at home or in the car. She is not at all comfortable in talking with her family about Tourette syndrome:

> I'm not. They are not comfortable with me. If I would bring it up, they would probably be like, "Oh, does that still bother you?" When I was younger and I went to all those doctors and got all that attention, I got really good at hiding it. Especially from my parents, because if they saw me doing it, then I would have to be on more sugar-free diets. (Stacy 79 – 82)

Likewise, she is not comfortable discussing Tourette with friends either:

> I don't. I'm rather uncomfortable. I wish I wasn't. (Stacy 84)

Stacy describes her own teaching style as fairly traditional:

> I'm relatively strict with the kids. I have pretty good classroom discipline. But I'm generally laid-back. I don't let them get away with a whole lot. I think I'm more laid back with my coworkers. I run a pretty tight classroom. They listen to me. They respect me. (Stacy 92 – 94)

Stacy does not feel like her Tourette affects her experiences with the community:

> I don't know if it really affects my involvement in the community. Sometimes I'm not as comfortable socializing. I'm not comfortable being around people all the time. I kind of need my alone time sometimes. But dating wise, not a whole lot. I was engaged for a while, and I told my ex about it, and he was really supportive. I could tic around him, and he wouldn't even notice. He was really cool about it. (Stacy 120 – 124)

She recalls being treated with kindness in elementary school because of having Tourette:

> They were really, really sensitive about it. Everybody was. I don't think anyone ever made fun of me. And my teachers were always really, really supportive. They all knew. I don't know if they talked about it with my parents, but maybe they were just good about explaining it to the kids. I don't know what they did because I didn't want to be there when they did it. Everyone was really supportive. Nobody ever made fun of me. I never lost any friends. I remember when I was on my crazy diet, my friends really helped me out with my diet. I had a little friend in third grade, and he would try to sneak me his Twinkie. (Stacy 171 – 177)

She did not think that people even noticed she had Tourette in high school because she concealed her tics:

> By that time, I had learned really well how to hide it. Everyone from elementary school had probably forgotten by then. And no one ever really knew. (Stacy 179 – 180)

Stacy's story portrays the life of an educator still in the early stages of her career. She does not feel comfortable talking to others about Tourette, so she conceals her tics. Because she has a mild case of Tourette syndrome, she is able to do this with success. This is not the norm. Many people with Tourette are able to suppress their tics for a short amount of time, but this is generally followed by a relief period in which a person tics more than usual.

Sue's Journey.

Sue is a 63 year old woman with Tourette syndrome. She taught middle school French for 33 years before retiring. She has a master's degree in French education. Sue had symptoms of Tourette syndrome long before she was diagnosed:

> It's interesting because I started with my symptoms when I was about six and a half, but I was not diagnosed until I was thirty six and a half. So it took a very, very long time for me to get my diagnosis. And, of course, that comes with a whole set of issues because nobody knew what was wrong. Like I said before, I think being in that small schoolhouse setting was a very good experience for me because it wasn't such a big issue. I also come from a large family of six children, and all of us had Tourette; none of us knew it. Because of the hereditary factor, my mom had it, so in the household it wasn't an issue. But nobody knew what it was, and my mother started when I was about six, six and a half, seven, started taking me to doctors to try to figure out what was going on, and obviously nobody had an answer because back then, they knew very little about it. And even 30 years later, they knew very little about it, so they gave me all kinds of diagnoses. I remember as a first grader, I was taken in to get glasses because I had a lot of eye blinking and eye scrunching. So they ended up referring me to an eye doctor, and I ended up getting bifocals at six years old. Which is totally ridiculous. Every time a new tic would start, they would have another reason for it. Like I was jerking my head back, and they told my mom it was because my bangs were too long, so she cut all my bangs off. These kind of silly things. And you know, after a while, you kind of just give up because you just really don't have an answer. And that's kind of what it has been. There were a lot of negative experiences with kids saying things, kids teasing, kids imitating. I guess I always knew that even though I knew I was different, I couldn't let it

stop me. That was just kind of my take on things. And so I just felt that I really needed to keep plugging away, and I was always, I guess, what I would probably call an overachiever. And probably because I wanted to be known for something besides the person who has these weird movements and tics and everything else. You know, that's not who I wanted to be known as, so I was always an overachiever. And I guess it's served me well. Throughout the years, I've done okay. But when I think back on all the negative experiences and as I grew into adulthood, I think that probably some of the good things that came out of that probably outweighed the bad because it has certainly made me a much more compassionate, empathetic, understanding teacher, no doubt about it. Because you know firsthand what it's like to grow up with some kind of a disorder that nobody understands, and so you really see that from that point of view with other kids. So that is a huge thing. And I think that's served me very well in life, I have to say. I really can't even remember specific incidences of things; I just know there was always a lot of, "Why are you doing this? Why do you keep doing that?" A lot of questions, a lot of teachers asking me to stop making noises and always trying to tell them that I really wanted to and I couldn't, but not being able to explain it. And I guess my thing, I always say this about kids with Tourette, I did not have the ADHD component. I have terrible OCD, and I have some learning disabilities, but I never had the ADHD, so I was not a problem child, as they look at kids with ADHD. And I think in some ways that was my saving grace. Because I was a strong student, I did very well academically in school, and I think that kind of saved me because they just figured, "Well, she obviously can't help what she's doing, but she's still achieving, and she's not causing any other problems in class," so they just kind of after a while, ignored it. And I think that was probably the best thing that happened. It was tough, I mean going from the one room schoolhouse with four kids in my class to a junior high with 25 kids in my class, was an issue. But we got through it. And in college what was probably the most difficult was taking notes; you know, I have dysgraphia, like a lot of people with Tourette do, and taking notes was always difficult for me. [Dysgraphia is a deficiency in the ability to write, mainly in terms of handwriting.] I have been blessed with a wonderful memory, which has served me very well in life, and I developed my own shorthand. I had my own little method of taking shorthand that I could do, so I could get the notes down. But it was a struggle, there's no question. But it worked for me because I always had, I guess sometimes, I always tell people, sometimes the OCD overrides. And when you're really obsessive about things, which I always was, it makes you that overachiever, and you spend three times as much time on something as anybody else does because you want to do it the best. And I think that was the OCD. So, in some ways, it was overriding everything else. So that was good in a lot of ways. (Sue 22 – 73)

She finally received her diagnosis 30 years later:

I was diagnosed when I was 36. I was home. It was a Sunday night, and I was trying to get all the school work I put off all weekend done. Because I hadn't done anything all weekend with my schoolwork. And I sat down in the chair in my living room, and I put my feet up on the footstool. And I got all my papers on my lap, and I started channel surfing to find something to watch. And there was a show that came on that you may not remember because you're young; it was called *Quincy*. The *Quincy* show, and it was actually *Quincy, M.E.* And he was a medical examiner or coroner, played by Jack Klugman, who was a real popular actor; it was quite a popular show back in the mid-80s. So I thought, "Well, this is a pretty good show; I'll watch this." So I started watching it, and he happened to be doing a story that night about a young boy with Tourette syndrome, and it was amazing. I had never even heard the words before, and as I was starting to watch it, I'm seeing this kid with all his movements and noises, and I'm thinking, "Wow, this looks a lot like what I do." I got no work done that night, as you can imagine because I was just spellbound by this program. And I didn't know it at the time, but that was probably the first show ever on in this country about Tourette. There had never been another show about Tourette. And I guess it was my good fortune to have been watching that night. At the end of the show, they put the name of our national Tourette Syndrome Association on the screen, and I called them the very next morning, before I even went to my homeroom. And back then, they had very little literature. That was 25 years ago. They had a couple little pamphlets. They sent them to me, and they also said they were going to send me the referral list for doctors in the state where I lived, that treated Tourette. And when I got the list, I was so disappointed because there were only two doctors on the whole list for the whole state. And I got an appointment, but it took me four months to see him. He was that busy. But I did go, and I did get my diagnosis. I also realized that, in that time that I was waiting to see him, that my whole family had this. I started thinking about it, and we all do this. I have three brothers and two sisters, and they all have tics, they have noises, a lot of the associated disorders. And by that time I had nieces and nephews, and a lot of them were showing signs of it, so I was aware at that time that it was a hereditary disorder, and we all had it. But I didn't honestly say anything to anyone until I was officially diagnosed. I didn't mention it even to my mom, who was alive at the time. I never said a word to her until after I was diagnosed. Because she had it herself and didn't know. She had had it for almost 60 years by the time she was diagnosed. That's kind of how the diagnosis took place. (Sue 92 – 125)

Sue wanted to become an educator because of her elementary school teacher:

I wanted to be a teacher from first grade. And I think it was probably my teacher that I had through all of elementary school. She was just wonderful. She was a fantastic lady. She just passed away a couple years ago actually, in her 90s. She was just one of those people that she saw it, she saw the tics, she heard the noises, but she just taught us with her heart. She was just a wonderful teacher, but I think now of my own classroom in comparison to her classroom. I mean six grades, all in one room. She had no telephone. She had no textbooks per se; we had a reading book, and we had a math book, and that was it. Everything had to be mimeographed, not copied, but everything had to be done with carbon paper. She had nobody else; you know I think of my classroom, and I could go down and talk to other adults in the staff room, and she had nobody but us. Not to have anybody else to consult with, to share things with; it was just really difficult. She was such a dedicated teacher that I think it was because of her that I, early on, I wanted to be a teacher. And I absolutely, never ever swayed from that path, ever. From the whole time I was growing up. When I got into high school, I knew that's what I wanted to do. When I started applying for colleges, I knew that's what I wanted to do, and I stuck with it. (Sue 75 – 90)

Sue reflects on the intellectual and emotional connections between her life and work and why she is the teacher she is:

I think I was probably and I don't know if I can really attribute this to having Tourette, but I was one of those teachers that, I wouldn't say I got overly emotionally involved, but I did get very involved with kids because I think I realized that everybody in life needs that one person. I know so many kids that will go to school in the morning, and not one teacher all day long gives them any special smile, special attention, gives them a special comment. And I think every kid needs that. I think they need somebody in their corner. And I felt if I had to be the one in their corner, I would be because I see these kids go through the day, some of them, with such problems, slow learners, and kids with all kinds of learning disabilities, and a lot of teachers aren't particularly accommodating to that and particularly understanding. So I felt that I had to be that one person who, when they walked in my room, I had to say something special to them. I used to try to stand in my classroom door every day before every class and as the kids came in, to say something to each kid. Whether it was a little joke or calling him a nickname just some little cute thing to let them know, you're safe in here. You can come in here and be safe, and you don't have to worry. And I think that's just so important. I think there is something that has to be said for that, the emotional aspect. Because having Tourette can be very emotional, let's face it. I know what it's like to have been teased and made fun of and kicked out of movie theaters and all these awful things. So I can relate to a lot of kids who deal with the same kind of things. And I think you do kind of get emotionally involved in it sometimes. (Sue 939 – 956)

As with many people with Tourette syndrome, Sue found it difficult to try to suppress her tics in order to conceal her disability:

Definitely, it's very hard to suppress. I mean you can do it, but it takes its toll. I know for a long time when people didn't know, I destroyed chairs in my house because I'd come home, and I have a lot of tics where I'd bang on things. And I would bang so hard on the chairs, I'd break the arms of them. It was from just trying to hold it in during the day. And I have some coprolalia. It's not as severe as some people's, and so as a teacher, not knowing what that was, it was really hard. It's not good for a teacher to be swearing at the kids. It's not appropriate. It was tough. You tried a lot of suppressing, going out into the hall, so it took its toll on me, I think, emotionally more than anything. (Sue 233 – 240)

Like many of the participants in this study, Sue was most comfortable ticcing at home alone.

Sue has felt the effects of discrimination when out in the community:

That's a tough one. I don't see any, I mean I guess years ago when I was first teaching, I was living in an apartment, and I had a lot of loud vocal tics. I had a tic where I would bang my head against the wall. And neighbors now and then would complain that I was making too much noise. And this was before I bought the house and before I knew what I had, so it was very hard to even give them an explanation. But that was a pretty rare occasion. It wasn't all that common. My vocal tics are noticeable, but they're not loud screaming kind of things like some people have. It wasn't all that bad. But for the most part, it wasn't that bad. You know there are certain places that I avoid. I really rarely go to the movies anymore because I have had a lot of problems in the movies. I honestly don't go to church anymore because you can't stop the church service, and people get annoyed because it's a quiet environment. I always say, "God understands." Libraries that are very quiet I may not spend a lot of time in. There are places that I avoid because of it, but that's my choice. It's just easier for me. You figure, when you're going somewhere, you're going there because you probably want to enjoy yourself, and how can you enjoy yourself when you're trying to suppress your symptoms? And you can't even pay attention to a movie you're watching or a book you're reading because all you're thinking about is what everyone else around you is thinking, so it's not fun. Sometimes it's just easier to stay home. (Sue 496 – 511)

Sue is very open to discussing Tourette syndrome with family members:

In my family, everybody has it. We were all diagnosed after I was diagnosed. We're pretty open about it. I have, I did have five brothers and sisters, one passed away, but every one of us have Tourette's. And I have a lot of nieces and nephews with it. We're pretty open about it. We joke about it a lot. You know, we have a good sense of humor about it, which has helped. I would say I'm pretty open. (Sue 268 – 272)

She also feels comfortable discussing Tourette with friends:

With friends I would say I'm fairly open. I think it depends. With close friends obviously they know, and it's not a big deal. It's become so much a part of what I do, running the chapter, and the book I just wrote, so people know about it. But casual acquaintances, casual friends, probably not so much. Any of my close friends, I have been very comfortable discussing it with them. (Sue 274 – 277)

A typical work day for Sue was filled with activity:

A rat race. My school started a little bit later than most; we didn't start until 9:00, so it wasn't a real early time. Prior to having medication for the OCD, it was a much different scenario because it was very hard on most mornings to get out of my house. I have a lot of OCD with straightening things, and symmetry and checking things and that kind of stuff. So it would take me a really long time, sometimes it would take me 25 to 30 minutes to get out of my house. And once I started taking medication for OCD, which didn't come until much later, it was a lot easier. I still have a lot of the symmetry and checking, but I could limit it much more so it didn't take me, I didn't have to go check that bedspread 10 times or the refrigerator to make sure the milk carton was straight and or whatever I had to do. So, that was always a challenge. But yet, because of the OCD, I always, I didn't start work until 9:00, and but for literally probably 20, 25 years of my career, I absolutely had to be in school no later than 7:30. And that was just my own OCD.

There is no reason I had to be there at 7:30, but in my head, I had to be there at 7:30. It was kind of like your brain is fighting you. You know you've got all of these things to check and make sure the heat is turned down and that this is turned off and all this kind of stuff and the symmetry, and yet you try to fight to get to school at a ridiculous time in which you didn't have to even be there at that time anyway. But once I started taking medication for the OCD, that was easier. And I have to say that it was also a lot easier because I knew I had Tourette, as I had an explanation to give people. I found myself many times, even when people knew, my whole life had been trying to suppress and camouflage. That was just my life. And not that I was totally successful because my tics are obvious, but I tried when I was at work, I would go into the bathroom and let the tics out there. Sometimes I knew if I had some cursing tics, I would go out into the hallway and do them then or into the garbage can. I think they always thought I was just a good hall monitor because I was out there checking on things. I was really out there swearing. Even after I was diagnosed, it's still something you tried to hide, especially the big stuff. But certainly I did it. And I always taught, because that I was a French teacher, I always taught six classes a day which was a very heavy schedule. Most people have five and then have a sixth non-teaching assignment, whether it be a study hall or cafeteria duty or whatever. I had six teaching assignments. Many times I had three, if not four, grade levels I was teaching in. So it made it very difficult because it's a lot of work. As an educator, when you have three or four different preparations, it's a lot of work to keep up with. And that was stressful for me, and, of course, stress makes the tics worse. So it was always a balancing act. But I think when we talked last week, I've always been one of those people, I don't want to be remembered for ticcing. And so I was an overachiever. I really worked, probably, much harder than most other teachers did. Which was necessary to keep up with everything I had to do. And still do other things, run clubs and whatever other activities I was running as extracurricular kind of stuff for school. It was a struggle, but you got through it. I think I've always been blessed with this great sense of humor. My whole family is that way. Even back when I didn't know, I could always find a way if the kids would say something to kind of laugh it off or get it to the point where they didn't even notice it anymore. I wanted them to get to know me as a teacher and respect me and like me as a teacher so that they wouldn't just notice the tics. And I think because I worked so hard at that, that I was successful at it. And now when I talk to former students, they say that all the time. They say, "You were fun, and you were creative, and you did great activities with us, and we just after a while stopped paying attention to it because we got to know you as a person. You didn't dwell on the tics, and that was just the way it was." But I think that's always in the back of your mind. It's like one more thing that a person with Tourette and OCD and some of the associated disorders has to do in addition to all the other things you have to do that are just part of being an educator, such as the daily working with the kids. I think that my day was very exhausting from trying to suppress symptoms to obsessing about everything to all the preparations and hiding things, and it was exhausting. But somehow you just keep up with it, and after a while, that's just your life. You don't know anything else. I taught, as I said, six classes. I was almost always after school for something, whether it was giving extra help to the kids, running the French club, I ran Student Council at our school for a lot of years, I always had some sort of activity going on, so it wasn't unusual for me to be there until 4:00 in the afternoon. And then come home and just collapse and tic your brains out. And get that all out of your system. And then start your school work for the next day. It was difficult. (Sue 286 – 340)

Sue describes her own teaching style as open, creative, and fun:

I try to establish a very friendly and very accepting classroom. That to me was the most important thing. The kids came in there, and they felt comfortable to talk to you about anything. And I think probably having Tourette was, this was one of the things that was really good about it, if I had to say there was something good about it. It made me always be a very nonjudgmental person. Kids could say anything to me, and it just didn't surprise me. I was just very nonjudgmental. I also wanted them to come into my classroom and feel safe. That was always a really key thing, that they felt safe. Like if you mess up, it's not the worst thing in the world. We'll discuss it, and we'll move on. I wasn't an overly strict disciplinarian, but I didn't have to be. Kids just didn't, I mean not that they didn't try things but more antics than anything. The chit chatting back and forth and stuff like that. When things like that happened, that's just a normal part of a classroom. I used to say, every now and then I'd say, "We'll have to start a talker's anonymous club for the kids who could not stop talking." They had to raise their hand and stand up and say, "My name is John, and I can't stop talking." Just be silly with things like that and find ways, find humorous ways, and ways that they then feel safe and that they were not being unduly disciplined. I also wanted it to be a fun class because I think that I realized this from some of the learning challenges that I had, that there are so many different learning styles. And most kids don't learn passively. Especially middle school kids. They learn actively. So it was always important to me to have a very active, everybody participating kind of classroom where everybody was involved in activities because the more you're involved in that, the better you're going to learn. And so we always had a game, we played Pictionary in French, we played Jeopardy, I made up songs that we would march to to learn different things. When we learned the days of the week, we'd march around the room and sing the days of the week. Stuff that kept the kids really, really involved and using a lot of music, even though I have absolutely no singing voice whatsoever. I think it was just that I wanted it to be a friendly, warm, comfortable, accepting, and safe classroom. And with a lot of different activities to kind of feed into everybody's learning style. If you could see a kid that really had a certain difficulty with a certain thing, well, find a different way to test them. Just about every test I gave, I had two versions. I had one with maybe fill in the blank for the average kid, and for the kid who had word retrieval problems, I had a word bank. And the kids never really knew this because they didn't know what the kid next to them had gotten. In middle school, you could pull that over on them. They don't catch on quite as much. I guess that's how I wanted my classroom to be, and when I see kids now, that's what I love that they say is, "We always loved your class because it was fun, but we learned so much having fun." One of the kids, I saw her recently, she is teaching at a school I just did a presentation at, and she said one time when I was teaching, "I remember one of the kids said, 'This is boring,' and you said, 'If you want boring, I can really show you boring. And then I remember everyone turning to the kid and saying, 'Ms. Clark is not boring.'" And I love hearing that because that's the kind of classroom I wanted. I think it's important for every kid, regardless of their disability, regardless of what makes them different, to walk into that room and feel safe. And feel like if somebody says something to them that's not appropriate that the teacher will put a quash to it. The teacher will not be reprimanding them or embarrassing them. I can honestly say to you that unless it was an absolute emergency situation, a kid throwing a desk across the room or whatever, that I never disciplined kids in front of other kids. I would always see them after class, have them come out into the hallway with me, I just wouldn't do that to them. It's the worst thing because kids have to save face. And if you discipline them in front of their friends, then you're just asking for them to try to save face. That's just the kind of teacher that I was. I think I became that kind of teacher, a lot of it because of the Tourette. Because I didn't know for so many years what I had, and a lot of this stuff happened to me. It does make you a much more empathetic person. (Sue 342 – 393)

She did use different strategies or accommodations that she made herself to deal with her Tourette in the classroom:

Yeah, I think the first strategy was just letting everybody know. It made me more comfortable, and it made the kids comfortable, so that was the easiest thing about it. The really difficult time for me was when there was any type of a quiet activity going on, which believe me, in middle school, there aren't that many. But every now and then, if you were giving a test that is lasting 40 minutes, or we'd have the state testing, and I'd have the kids in there for a couple of hours, I was always afraid that my noises were disturbing them. So that was one thing that was really hard for me. And what I used to do was when my students were taking tests, I always had a tape deck or a CD player or something on my desk, and I would play French music. Because I was teaching French, and I would tell them that it really will help you, by osmosis, if you hear French music and you're taking a French test, you'll do better. What I was really doing was camouflaging my noises. That was my trick; I'd sit at my desk or somewhere near the tape deck, so they couldn't hear me. And it did make a big difference. It really did. So little things like that. I learned to sometimes turn to the blackboard to try to say the curse word without people hearing it or to try to muffle it, so yeah, I learned some strategies over the years. Although my students did say they heard me say the words. And I would say, "Darn it. I thought I was being so careful." I never asked for accommodations, but I did make many on my own. Lots of turning to the blackboard or going out to the hall when I knew I had to swear. Doing tons of my work on the computer because I knew my handwriting has always been a real issue. Earlier on it was not so easy because we didn't have computers, that's how old I am, when I first started teaching. There wasn't an opportunity, so it was hard. I definitely, along the way, made a lot of my own accommodations. I figured out when I needed to take breaks, finding places to go where I could take the breaks. But I've never asked for any. On another note, I have gone into schools on behalf of teachers with Tourette and/or OCD and helped them get accommodations. And the schools that I have gone into have been quite good about it. (Sue 243 – 257, 567 – 575)

Sue reflects on her treatment in elementary school by teachers and peers because of having Tourette:

Elementary school, I think I mentioned earlier I went to a one-room schoolhouse in the mountains for six years, and I had the same teacher. And my sisters and brothers were all in the school with me, and so it was just never an issue with her because, I knew she knew something was wrong, probably wondered. It was just never brought up, never ever an issue. The only time I ever remember my teacher ever saying anything was when I had a real bad eye blinking tic when I started, it was the first tic I had, and I was the second oldest in my family but the first one to start with tics, and I remember she talked to my mom and suggested that I go to the eye doctor. Because she thought I was having vision problems. But after that, it was just never mentioned again. We never heard any more about it. Now when I was in middle school or junior high as we called it, and I transferred because the one-room schoolhouse ended, and we had to go into a school in town and my mother put me in a parochial school, that was a little harder because I was now the only one in my class with Tourette and the nuns were a little strict. But, I was a pretty strong student and that helped. And the other thing that helped a lot, I think if I had gone to the public school it might've been more difficult, is that my aunt was a nun at the school, and she was one of the beloved ones. Everybody loved my aunt. And so, knowing that we were the nieces and nephews really helped a lot. And she kind of had our back. But it was definitely more difficult in middle and high school because you got questioned about it more, people would tell you to stop doing things, and you couldn't help it. I had never experienced that before because in my little one-room schoolhouse, the unreal world, my non reality world, it really was not an issue. So why do these people care all of a sudden why I'm doing these things? So it did become much more difficult. Definitely. (Sue 970 – 991)

Her Tourette syndrome became a little bit more of an issue in high school:

I think the same thing, it became more of an issue. I think probably one of my saving graces was I was a strong student. And I definitely feel badly for some of these kids that have really bad ADHD, have some learning disabilities because they're not doing well in school, so it just adds to that whole attitude that teachers have about them. They don't care, they are irresponsible, that kind of thing. I was never looked at as that. If anything, it was when I went into the junior high and all the way through most of high school, my OCD got really, really bad. I was this horrible perfectionist who would copy things over and over, and everything had to be just so, and I was a model student. Because I had perfect work because I would spend hours doing it. I was a model student, so I had these things going on, but it wasn't a huge issue. But I don't see that a lot with kids who have really bad learning disabilities and ADHD or some of the other issues that go along with Tourette. It makes it much more difficult for them. I was lucky that I could be a strong student and a shining star, as well as having Tourette. That really helped me a lot because I know with my sister, my one sister that passed away, had Tourette,

ADHD, terrible OCD, depression disorder, and she also had an 80 percent hearing loss. And nobody cared that you had these problems back then. She just struggled through school. And she didn't end up going back to get her degree until she was in her mid-40s. She went back and got her bachelor's and her master's degree. Because nobody helped her with anything. Oh, you have a hearing loss? Well alphabetically, she's in the back, so there we go. Nobody cares. I think one of the things that I had going for me was the fact that I was a strong student. And so it became less of an issue, but it was still there. Definitely. (Sue 993 – 1012)

Sue also reflects back on her life in college. She believes she was treated differently in college, but many times, she was oblivious to it:

I mean people would say things to me all the time about it, but I didn't know what it was. As a matter of fact, it is interesting, we just had a reunion. I was a French major, and we decided to have a reunion of the, at the time it was an all-girls' school, now it's a coed school, and we had 12 of us who went on to study for a year in France. And we all took a ship over together and lived in dorms together. Incredibly close. Over the years after we graduated, we lost track of each other, and we had a reunion last summer. It was just fantastic. Some of these kids I hadn't seen in 40 years. And everybody brought up the Tourette. Everybody. I guess I never thought about it when I was with them. But they said things like, "We always knew there was something. We never knew what it was." And then my former roommate, who was a roommate for three years when I was in college said, "Sometimes you used to drive me totally crazy with this and many other things, but you were a nice person. We loved you. We just didn't say anything, but yeah, we did notice it definitely." And they were all so supportive of all the work that I have done, and they said, "You don't realize this, but we follow you on Facebook. We follow you on the Internet," because I'm so involved in everything, and I just wrote a book that's being published this month, so they all knew about all this stuff. These are people I haven't seen in 40 years. So it's nice to see that even though it was an issue, they were very kind to me. Nobody ever said too much about it. Some of my friends suggested maybe I should try to see different doctors. And I remember saying to them, "I've been doing that for years. Nobody knows what this is. So I've given up on it. What's the point in going to 20 more doctors? What's the point of it?" And it was interesting to see, so many years later, what they all said. Yes, they did notice, and yes, they did worry and wonder, but now for the last many years, they've been following all my work and everything that I'm doing. (Sue 1014 – 1035)

It meant so much to her that her friends wondered and worried about her but that they also looked past it because they loved her for who she was:

That was huge for me. That was a huge thing. It really, really was. One of the girls said, "I can't believe how incredibly brave you were." She said, "If I had had this, and especially not knowing what it was. Here you are, 19 years old and putting yourself on a ship and going to Europe to live in France for a year. God, you think they knew about it in the United States, they certainly didn't know about it in France. And you just did it." And I said, "Well, I think I just decided early on that I don't care what this is, I'm going to do what I want to do. I'm not going to let this stop me. I can do it. Why can't I do it?" And I think that's always been my attitude. (Sue 1038 – 1045)

She believes her treatment in school because of having Tourette did have an influence on her wanting to become an educator:

> Yeah, I think so. I think so. And that's probably more elementary school. Because my elementary teacher was so kind and so caring and so nurturing in so many ways that it did. From very early on, I decided I wanted to be a teacher. That's what I wanted to do. And I think probably part of it was because of her level of caring, nurturing, and empathy, despite everything. She just seemed to have that. And it really made me want to be a teacher. Definitely. I never swayed from that. From six years old all the way through high school, anytime people said to me, "What do you want to be?" I told them, "A teacher. That's what I want to do. It's what I want to do." I never changed my mind. (Sue 1048 – 1055)

Sue's story portrays the life of a veteran teacher with Tourette syndrome. Sue's ability to be successful despite anything that life throws at her is seen throughout her life of being an educator for 33 years. She has numerous stories, all of which are exemplary of a successful teacher. Sue was a role model for thousands of students and is a role model for all teachers, not just teachers with a disability.

Conclusion

The participants in my study are seven educators with Tourette syndrome from six different states across the country. They range from a teacher who just completed her first year in the profession to an educator who retired after 33 years of teaching. Although there are difficulties in being a teacher with a disability, these educators demonstrate that it is possible to persevere in life and overcome one's disability in order to be a successful educator. These seven educators are evidence that teachers with a disability are a contribution, even an asset, to school districts. It is my hope that my portrayal of these seven educators will encourage administrators to actively recruit educators with disabilities for their school districts.

CHAPTER FIVE

DISCLOSING TO ADMINISTRATORS AND COLLEAGUES

Purpose

In this chapter, I will discuss participants' decisions on whether or not to disclose their disability to administrators and colleagues. In looking at disclosing to administrators and colleagues, I focused on three main questions: 1) Do you disclose to administrators and colleagues? 2) Have you ever tried not to disclose at work? 3) How does Tourette syndrome shape your relationships with other faculty?

When focusing on these three questions, ten main themes emerged. These included: 1) disclosing during the interview process, 2) disclosing to colleagues, 3) disclosing to administrators, 4) suppressing tics to hide one's disability, 5) the comfort level in discussing Tourette syndrome with others at work, 6) how disclosing impacted relationships with colleagues, 7) positive experiences due to disclosing at work, 8) challenges experienced due to disclosing at work, 9) discrimination faced due to disclosing, and 10) socialization with colleagues outside of work.

Disclosing During the Interview Process

Not all of the participants knew they had Tourette syndrome when they first began their teaching careers. This influenced whether they disclosed in the interviewing process or not. Of the three participants who knew they had Tourette when they

110

began interviewing, two of them disclosed in the interviewing process.

Laura was not sure about whether to disclose in the interview process or not. She ended up disclosing in some interviews but not others. Disclosing did not seem to hamper her, as the first interview she disclosed in was the job she was offered:

> I was kind of hesitant, I was like, I don't know if I should tell my interviewers that I have Tourette's, but at the same time, I don't want them to see me blinking all funny and think that I'm not taking this seriously or just doing something goofy. And so I decided that I would tell them if it became an issue during the interview. And I had a couple of interviews, and it was never an issue, so I didn't actually bring it up. And then the school where I got hired to teach fifth grade, they actually asked me, "How will we know when you're stressed?" And I thought to myself, well, I guess I should tell them and said, "My Tourette's gets bad." And they were just like, "Okay." And we just kind of moved on. I was like, "Whoa, that was weird. They don't care." (Laura 50 – 58)

Laura interviewed at the end of her first school year for a different job in the same district. Although the district already knew she has Tourette syndrome, she did not disclose in this interview:

> The district knows about my disability. I don't think that my administrators at the middle school know. And it's not that I plan on keeping it a secret, there was just not an opportunity to tell them during the interview that I had. (Laura 106 – 108)

Tracey was extremely open to disclosing about Tourette syndrome at the very start of her career. She started in her job interviews:

> I did actually. I was part of the Tourette's Association, so it was on my resume that I volunteered there. No one ever questioned it. I think my current school asked me how I felt that it made me a good educator. And my answer to them was I felt that because I have a disability, I know how to be patient and understanding to those children with a disability. (Tracey 69 -72)

Mike's condition of Tourette's Syndrome is more severe, so to him, there was no hiding it in job interviews. He was open and forthright from the beginning:

> When I started looking for jobs, interview after interview, I couldn't get the principal to hire me. As an elementary schoolteacher, a lot of them said that they wouldn't hire me because I had Tourette's syndrome. They said that, "How could you possibly be effective in the classroom making all those noises?" They said, "How are we going to educate our parents, our students, our community?" I said, "Be open and honest. We'll educate them, we'll get through it." At that time, I had a lot of self-confidence. I had a lot of great experiences in college and high school, and I had no reason to believe I couldn't be an effective teacher. I had great student teaching experiences. I was ready to do it, I just couldn't find somebody to believe in me. I even had one principal state, "If you worked in my school, the students would beat you up." And I said, "We'll educate them." And that's what I tried to do, but no one wanted to listen. So interview after interview, I couldn't get a job. You know, it was definitely a part of my journey. I considered, maybe

I do need to give up, maybe I need to find something else, but deep down, deep down I knew that this was what I'd be good at doing. I didn't want other people to get the best of me. I tried to keep that positive attitude, definitely kept the perseverance, didn't want to make excuses. I was just driven to do it, I have that passion for education and just making a difference. And then there was an opportunity, when I interviewed, my 25th interview, and on that interview, it was an interview like no other I'd ever had before. They started asking questions like, "What is your philosophy of education? What's your classroom management style? How do you communicate with parents? How do you do reading? How do you do math?" And the other 24 interviews really didn't ask those questions. They could only focus on me being a guy who had Tourette's syndrome. I continued that conversation, and before I left that day, they hired me as a second grade teacher. And I was able to fulfill my dream of being that teacher. I took on the responsibility, and I knew what my first lesson was going to be, it was going to be about educating kids. That just because you're different, if you have a disability in life or a weakness in life, you can overcome your challenges, just like I was able to overcome mine. And that you can fulfill your dreams, like I was able to. (Mike 55 – 80)

Mike again mentioned there was nothing he could hide in his job interviews:

I couldn't hide it, there's nothing to hide. Out of the 25 interviews that I went on to become a teacher, there was one interview that I went on that I decided I was going to try not to share. And I tried it, and it was too uncomfortable. It wasn't who I am. I'm this person who's always been open and honest.

That's just who I am, it's how I deal with it. That's how I've overcome my challenges. So, the whole interview, I didn't feel, I wasn't me. So I decided that's not how I do it. I'm going to be open and honest, and if they can't accept me for who I am, then I don't need them. Truly, if they couldn't support me and understand my condition in an interview, and how are they going to support me being an educator when parents start asking questions or kids start asking questions? I knew that I just needed a supportive administrator, and it was a great way to find out if I had their support. (Mike 108 – 117)

Stacy, unlike the others, has never disclosed in any job interviews. She is not yet comfortable discussing Tourette syndrome in her professional world. Similar to Stacy, I did not disclose in job interviews when I began interviewing either.

Disclosing to Colleagues

Even if participants disclosed initially during their interviews, they would all have to decide if and when they were going to disclose to their colleagues. Most of the participants did disclose to some degree while teaching. Some disclosed openly once they were diagnosed; others disclosed to those they were closest to or on a need-to-know basis.

After Laura started her first job last year, she did disclose to her colleagues after talking with her mentor:

At first I didn't tell my colleagues because I didn't want to be seen differently, I just wanted to be viewed as an equal. But people started to talk, and I heard some things going around, and finally my mentor told me, "You know, people are asking me questions, and I really think it would just be better coming from you." So if I was talking to someone and I started ticcing a lot, I would tell them, "Oh sorry, I have Tourette's." And most of the time they were just like, "Oh okay." Some of them had questions about it or whatever, but they were fine with it. (Laura 110 – 115)

Michelle's story of disclosing at work is a little different because when she started working, she did not know that she had Tourette syndrome. She knew she had tics, but she didn't know the name for the condition. After she found out she had Tourette, she did start disclosing, but not right away. People have to be ready to be out and open and willing to discuss Tourette; until then, people usually try to suppress or just avoid discussing the situation. Even if it is apparent that they have some sort of medical condition, people with Tourette cannot discuss it with others until they are comfortable with it themselves:

Not right away. In the beginning, I guess the job I have now I knew. But I really didn't, I don't know, I work so hard on hiding it all the time just because. Even now, I'll try to be more comfortable ticcing, especially with my kids. Because we tell them they should tic. And we go to this wonderful camp that they have for kids with Tourette's. It's every October. And the whole camp is ticcing. It's the perfect place. I can totally relax and tic there. But for some reason, it's just really hard for me to let myself tic. I don't know, I guess just because it's so ingrained in me after all these years. So I think I just really never did mention it because it was really a non-issue. But I am noticing at work now that the more that I do talk about it, because everybody that I work with knows that my kids have it, we're always fundraising for them, and I think that the more that I talk about my kids having it, people ask questions, we're really open about it, I'm more comfortable ticcing now. And now, certain teachers know, I guess the ones I have lunch with, they'll know what tics I have. And this is so stupid but, in my house, we'll tic to make each other tic. I don't know. We're kind of goofy that way. But you have to laugh. You live with Tourette's, you have to laugh. My husband has allergies so he sniffs, so then I have to sniff. Then my daughter has to sniff. Then my husband sniffs again. And it's just funny. That's an example of, there's a teacher at work who, she was sniffing. And I'm like, "You are killing me. That is one of my tics." So now the more people who know about it, they're becoming more aware of it, and I'm not hiding it as much. This is the first year, the school year just ended, but this is the first school year that, and I've told this to many people, I didn't face my desk towards the door. And I've always faced my desk towards the door, so that I'll see someone as they come in because if I'm ticcing, and someone walked in, I would stop. So now, it doesn't face the door, and I said that to a lot of people, that is really big for me. So I could be in the middle of a facial tic and somebody could walk in, and it's okay. I'm just getting more used to it, I guess. (Michelle 82 – 105)

Similarly, her colleagues were supportive as well:

They were completely surprised but very open about it, very accepting about it, just really surprised. They had no idea. (Michelle 154 – 155)

Michelle understood that they were surprised because she has always worked at hiding her tics:

And I'm really good at, that I'll tic, but I'll tic so little that unless you know what I'm doing, you'll not necessarily see it. I'll tic under the table or I'll tic just enough that I feel it, and then I don't tic anymore. So when they found out they were like, "No way, I never saw you tic." And I'm like, "I'm ticcing right now, you just don't see it." But they were surprised. (Michelle 158 – 161)

Like Michelle, Jason also discovered he had Tourette syndrome after he was already working. Like many, he was not too sure about disclosing at first:

No I did not. Like I said, whenever I found out at the doctor, I was, at the time, my dates are horrible, I think it was in 2005. I did tell my building coordinator. She's kind of like a principal but she wasn't, that I had it because they were going to send me to a conference about Tourette's syndrome. I thought a couple of kids that I had might have had it, but their other disabilities is what was more of their thing. But they had the yelling out loud and coughing and the touching stuff a lot like the obsessive compulsiveness and that's why I wanted to go. And she's like, "Well, why would you want to go to that?" I said, "Well, I actually think I have it." And she's like, "Oh." She never did say anything else about that. When it kind of came out to my colleagues is when I was at another school. I had told just a few of the sixth-grade teachers that I worked with that I had it. And they were cool with it. I told them it was a mild case, and I don't cuss or anything like that, and they were fine with it. And they went and ran some races with me. I was a runner, so I ran with team TSA. We got a new principal that year, and I went that whole year, and my second year, I had a student who definitely had Tourette's syndrome. And of course, I was the first one to realize it. A lot of them kept thinking, "Why is this kid making these noises in class?" And I'm like, "Well, this is what I think." And they were like, "Oh, well that makes sense." How it came out to my corporation that I had Tourette's syndrome was the boy that had TS, he went in a study hall room, and they had a sub, substitute teacher. And the substitute teacher, I guess, was really harassing that kid because he was making noises, and she kept telling him to be quiet and blah blah blah. And it really upset the boy, and I guess he had told his mother about it, and his mother was just irate. And I was good friends with that boy and the mother because of our tie. I had actually told that mother about me, that I had it, and I talked to the boy and everything. So she had called the administration building, and she was trying to get the sub fired because of the way she treated that boy in class. She told the superintendent, "Well, Mr. Marks's been helping us out with the situation because he has Tourette's." And they didn't even notice. They were like, "Oh, well we didn't know that." But they never did say anything about it. (Jason 97 – 123)

At the start, Jason was disclosing only on a need-to-know basis:

Just that one building coordinator, I had told her. And just my close colleagues. When I get to know people, I tell them. I just don't run up and start a job and say I have Tourette's. Like when I go to my new elementary this year in fifth grade, I'm not just going to go tell everybody that, but once I get closer to people, I'll let them know. Or if they start to notice. I've had a couple students, I did a mentoring program last year, I was a sub mentor. I had a couple kids keep staring at me and giggling because I was rolling my eyes and making my eyebrows do something weird and they're like, "What are you doing that for?" I did tell them, and I knew I wasn't going to have those kids anymore because I was leaving schools. I told them what it was, and of course they didn't understand. They were fifth-graders. So I just kind of blew that off because that's how they are. But once I got to know people, my first year at my last school, like I said, I had only told one lady that I had it, and she and her husband, the first year, are the ones who ran that race with me. The second year is when I got to know a lot of other people, my colleagues, and that's when I started letting them know. (Jason 149 – 161)

Once he did start disclosing to colleagues, they were supportive:

They were fine with it. They were like everyone else and said, "Well, I've never noticed it" and I'm like, "Well, most people don't because I'm pretty good at hiding it." It comes out at night, and my wife notices it now. I tic a lot at home. I think it's years of holding in my tics around people until I get around the corner or whatever. They just don't really notice it, but the more comfortable I get with people, the easier it is to let a little tic out here or there slightly. But they're all fine with it. (Jason 179 – 184)

He is more comfortable discussing Tourette with people at work than he has ever been before, although he does not feel comfortable initiating the conversation:

I'm fine with it now. Like I said, if people had questions about it, I was fine answering them. As far as coming out and saying it, I'm not comfortable just saying I have it. But when the situation arises like with that boy, I was fine with it. I was fine discussing it with whoever wanted to talk about it. (Jason 233 – 236)

Everyone was accepting of Tracey at work:

> My colleagues were very supportive. They have never said anything negative about it. I was [teaching] in fifth grade at that point, but I was also young going into teaching. I was I think 26, 25, something like that when I got my job. They were very understanding and took me under their wing. (Tracey 75 – 78)

Sue's condition was apparent for many years before she was diagnosed with Tourette syndrome. As she worked at the same school district for her entire career, they knew she had some sort of condition, although no one ever knew what it was. However, once she was diagnosed, she did start disclosing, a little bit at a time:

> After I was diagnosed, I started telling a few friends. And, of course, everybody had noticed all these things, but nobody really knew. And then after a while, I just became, because I was starting a chapter, articles were in the newspaper. They had the big article about me in one of our local newspapers, and everybody saw it, and I think it just started becoming known. Once I knew, I was always very open about talking about it. I've never shied away from talking about it. Because I think I spent 30 years trying to figure this out, and I look at my family and what a lot of them have gone through because of nobody knowing over the years. To me, education is the key. That's the bottom line. And if we can educate people and talk about it, I'm in the perfect position to do that; I was an educator. And, so to me, it was fine. (Sue 142 – 150)

Once she knew that her condition was called Tourette syndrome, she was very open about it.

Sue's colleagues and friends were also supportive:

They were very supportive, I have to say. Everybody that I knew, all my friends were like, "Wow, what a neat thing," because everybody noticed it, and people have asked about it, but my answer was always, "I don't know." I've tried for years to find out why I do these things, and sometimes I'd make stuff up because I didn't have any idea what it is, but I didn't have an answer. And I think they were just so happy to know that finally I had an answer to my problem. You know, they could feel better. (Sue 200 – 205)

Stacy does not disclose at work. She wishes she were more comfortable discussing Tourette, but right now, she is not.

Disclosing to Administrators

Similar to deciding whether or not to disclose to their colleagues, participants had to decide whether or not to disclose to their administrators. Michelle noted that once she started disclosing at work, her administrators were supportive:

They were totally unfazed. It didn't faze them at all. As a matter of fact, I'm part of the, our school has a child study team. Where if the teacher has a difficult time with a student and they don't know what to do, they'll bring it up to us. We have meetings once a week. So there's myself, the psychologist, the social worker, a special ed teacher, all the experts, they call us, in the building. Anytime there's any kid who they're just not sure, you know if it looks like obsessive compulsive disorder. Does it look like maybe he has tics or something? Right away they're like okay, Mrs. Browning is going to go up and observe the kid. She's going to hang out in the classroom for a while. So it's kind of nice. Because they do, they take advantage of the fact that when it comes to Tourette's, I probably am the expert in the building. So they really have been really great about it. (Michelle 143 -152)

Eventually, it became common knowledge that Jason had Tourette syndrome, but it was disclosed after he had been there a while:

Yeah, and of course my principal, he has no sense of privacy or anything. He started telling everybody, "Well, Jason has Tourette's." And I'm like, "Thanks for telling everybody." But I didn't care at that point. I thought whatever. I'm fine with it now. But, when I first found out, in 2005, I was pretty secretive. I'd barely even told my in-laws or parents. (Jason 126 – 129)

His principal did not make a big deal out of the knowledge that Jason had Tourette syndrome:

He didn't say much. Like I said, I hate to say this, but he's kind of a self-absorbed kind of guy. He has shoulder shrugs and he said, "Well, maybe that's what I've got." I'm like, "Well, it's more than just shrugging your shoulders, it is a combination of things." He didn't say much. And he's an older guy, he's been doing that for 40 years. That was my fear all along. It wasn't so much the principal, it was when the administration caught wind of it. When the superintendent had called me, he had said, "Jason, this lady had called me. It was the mother of that kid, and she was complaining about the sub. And she had told us that you have Tourette's." And I'm like, "Yes sir, that's true." So he said, "Well, I was wondering if you could help handle the situation with the mother." I said, "Yeah, I don't mind at all." That was the last I ever heard of it. So as far as discrimination, I've not had any of that. And I was scared with this school corporation because of that, I really was. Because we have a lot of old-school school board members, a lot of old-school teachers, and I'm thinking, "Oh no." But I've not seen it. I was really happy about that. Whenever he called me I thought, "Well, he's okay with it. Cool." (Jason 163 – 177)

Jason feels empowered by disclosing at work because he knows that his superintendent is willing to call on him for assistance in working with other students or situations in the school district.

Tracey's principal was unfazed:

They were fine. My boss is an amazing principal, and she is just very understanding. It's never actually been brought up in meetings or anything. The only time we ever had an issue was when I had a parent complain about it, and even then, she was very supportive. (Tracey 80 – 82)

Once he got hired, Mike's administration was extremely supportive:

They embraced me 110 percent. I think their attitude was: we work with kids every day that have special needs. We tell these kids they can be anybody they want. They can do anything they want. They can follow their dreams. And ultimately, our administrators decided if we're going to talk the talk, then we need to walk the walk. Later on, when they talked to me about the interview and what they saw in me and how I eventually got to where I was, the talk was, "This is the candidate." I guess they score you on a one to five level, and with the county, I got five. They said, "You know, this guy is a five, but he's got

Tourette's syndrome." My administrator said, "Okay, so. And he's a five?" They responded, "Yeah." They told me that, that shows that they really wanted to take the journey with me. My administrator is definitely special. They embraced me till the end. They supported me. If a parent had a problem with it, they tackled it straight on. They did what they had to do. So, yes, they very much embraced me. (Mike 120 – 130)

When Sue started disclosing, her administration was supportive:

Well, you know, at that time I had already been teaching 15 years. And I had established my reputation in the building. I had tenure, and so they were extremely supportive of everything I was trying to do to get a chapter going. As a matter of fact, they let me use our school building for meetings. We had our support group meetings there; we had our kids' group there, conferences there. We used the auditorium. They were very supportive. Because I think they realized that it was, and not only that but I became the contact person. I taught at a very large school district with about 12 schools, three high schools, four middle schools, a lot of elementary schools. And so I became kind of their key contact person when they had somebody else in the district diagnosed with Tourette syndrome. They would immediately call me to go over and meet with teachers. And so they were using and abusing me, so they had to be nice to me. So that worked, and it was kind of a win-win situation. (Sue 174 – 184)

Suppressing Tics to Hide One's Disability

Many people with Tourette syndrome have tried at various times to suppress their tics in order to hide their disability. Different people have varying degrees of success with this. Like many people with Tourette syndrome, Laura found it difficult to suppress her tics when she had not disclosed and was trying to hide her condition:

> Oh yes. It seems like as soon as I told someone about it, it was so much less. I think that's just the anxiety. Because it gets worse when I get anxious. So I'm afraid people are noticing, and then it gets worse. If they already know, I don't really care. (Laura 141 – 143)

Because Michelle's Tourette's is a milder case, she did not find it as difficult to suppress her tics before she started disclosing:

> Not really. I think the hardest time was when I would be alone in my room. The whole moving my desk to a different place. Because I don't think much about it when I have a group of students, and I'm involved in doing something else. It's more when I'm alone and doing paperwork that it really hits me. So I guess at the beginning, when I was alone in my room and my desk wasn't facing the door, that was hard because I was always conscious of if someone was going to walk in. But as the school year has gone on, that hasn't been a problem. And now if they walk in and I'm making a face, they walk in and I'm making a face. As a matter of fact, I was coming out of the computer lab or something, and I'll open the door, and there's a teacher there and I'm in the middle of the face things, I'll be like, "Oh, you just caught me ticcing."

And they're like, "I did, I didn't even notice."
Because they don't notice. (Michelle 174 – 183)

Jason, like many with Tourette syndrome, found it more difficult to suppress his tics when he was not out and open about having Tourette:

> Yeah, I do. Because I notice it, this is not education related, but at movies or ballgames I hear people whisper or snicker whenever I'm shaking my head or constantly jerking my neck or something. Just because again, they don't know that I have it. And I try to hold it in. It's harder when you're trying to hold it in; it's harder. I think it's like coprolalia, where they cuss, they say they know they don't want to say the word and they know they shouldn't say the word, but they're in a situation where they just say it. And that's like when my neck tics hard when I'm at a ball game or something. I know I don't want to do it because no one knows what it is and that I have it, so it makes it a little bit harder to hold it in. (Jason 204 – 211)

Tracey does find it difficult to suppress her tics if she has not disclosed to someone:

> Yes, because growing up, I did not like to talk about it. And even now in an environment, you don't always bring it up. And I do find that it's hard because you want to do these head movements or the arm jerks and you're trying to stop yourself, and I feel like you focus so much on that, that you're not paying attention to what's going on around you. (Tracey 132 – 135)

Stacy feels like the older she gets, she does a better job of ticcing when no one is looking. As I did not disclose my disability when I began teaching, I tried to suppress my tics at work. I was not successful at this, as students and colleagues did notice. I believe people knew I had something, although they may have not known what it was.

Comfort Level in Discussing Tourette Syndrome with Others at Work

Comfort levels vary in discussing Tourette syndrome with people at work. Even though some people disclose at work, conversations about Tourette are not always easy. Although Laura has disclosed at work, it is not always easy talking to people about Tourette:

> It's easier than talking to my family because there's not that ashamed feeling. They don't feel responsible for it. It's easier, of course, to tell people that I'm closer to at work. It just depends on the person. Well, I get really embarrassed sometimes about it. And so a lot of times, I won't want to go to happy hour after school or to a Christmas party or something. I get really anxious about going because I don't want people to notice my tics. And they tend to get bad in social situations because I'm really introverted. So it's frustrating because I felt like people were always looking at my tics instead of listening to what I was saying. But then when I would be like, "I'm sorry." I always apologize for it. "I'm so sorry, my Tourette's is really bad right now." They'd all be like, "Oh, we're used to it. Don't even worry about it." So really it was all inside my head. I get a complex about it sometimes. (Laura 163 – 165, 211 – 218)

Now that Michelle has been disclosing at work, she is finding it easier and easier to discuss Tourette syndrome with her colleagues:

Well, I guess I would say I'm much more comfortable now. I would always talk about it in terms of my kids. Like that, I've always been really comfortable, talking about them. Over the last year or year and a half, I'm much more comfortable talking about it in reference to myself. (Michelle 200 – 202)

Tracey, because of experience, has become comfortable discussing Tourette syndrome with others:

I think I'm comfortable with that. I mean if they ask questions about it, I have no problem telling them about it. I definitely think I go out of my way more and more. I remember in college, there was this one guy who was making a comment, he was making a negative comment about Tourette's. And I remember very unlike myself, I just piped in and raised my hand, and I told the professor, "Well I have it, and I disagree with what this guy is trying to say." And I feel like since then, you have to kind of be more comfortable discussing it because people don't understand. They feel like it's, you know, if you see a movie where they're making fun of it, I think people just kind of feel like that's what it is, the verbal swearing. They don't realize how much more in-depth it is. (Tracey 154 – 162)

Mike is comfortable talking with colleagues about Tourette's:

Yes. You've got to be open and honest, and then I realize it's the same for my relationship skills, my openness. It was what my character was really built on. And I think that's what they appreciated about me. That I'm not going to hide this condition, and I'm not going to make excuses for this. This is who I am. And that's just what it is. (Mike 177 – 180)

The better Sue knew a colleague, the more comfortable she felt discussing Tourette syndrome with that person:

> Well, once I was diagnosed and it took a long time to have that happen, I was comfortable with close colleagues, but there were some people in the building that I still felt weren't as knowledgeable about it. So you didn't feel as comfortable discussing it. With people that I worked with for a long time or colleagues of mine, I was very comfortable. Very comfortable. There were certain people you just didn't talk to about it too much because they probably didn't really understand. (Sue 279 – 284)

Stacy thinks she would feel comfortable discussing Tourette if someone asked her a direct question about it, but she is not comfortable initiating these conversations:

> If somebody asked me questions, I would happily answer them and give them information. But nobody really does. Unless it is like someone I am dating. And oddly enough, every time I date, if I'm on a date, for instance I was on a date with this guy who was watching a basketball game or something and he kept shouting like, "Ball, ball, ball." He was watching this basketball game and he said, "Sorry, you probably think I have Tourette's." He had no clue that I had Tourette's. Usually they don't until they start making fun of people with Tourette's and I'm like, "Hey now. Let's talk about this." (Stacy 111 – 117)

For many years, I was not comfortable discussing Tourette syndrome with people at work. In fact, I did not talk about it openly until I began writing about it.

How Disclosing Impacted Relationships with Colleagues

Disclosing or not disclosing at work can impact one's relationships with colleagues. Laura has learned that being open about her Tourette forces her to talk about it, even when she feels self-conscious:

> That one's a little bit harder because with people my own age, I always feel a little bit more judgmental. It is, once people find out about it, they're usually pretty cool about it, and they're just like, "Whatever." It does make me have to be able to talk to people about hard things. And just be able to be really honest. (Laura 303 – 306)

Michelle feels that Tourette syndrome has impacted her relationship with other faculty and staff, but not in a bad way:

> I don't think it impacted in a bad way. Now that they know, I think it's kind of cool that they know and that they have somebody to go to if they have questions about a particular kiddo in their class. And I think we laugh about it, a lot, in my life. Whether it's at home or whatever. So if I'm in the classroom, in my room, for example, and someone walks in and catches me in a tic, it's funny. I always joke about it. Like, "Augh, you caught me making that face," or whatever. I don't think it really has impacted them in a bad way at all. And it's nice because people, they know that, even before they knew that I had it, they knew that my kids had it. And I was always very open to talk about it, so they just know that they can ask me any questions at all. (Michelle 239 – 246)

Jason does not feel like Tourette has a big impact on his relationships with colleagues at work:

I don't think it really does. Well I guess like I said that guy who had whispered that to the other colleague, "How does a guy with Tourette's not tic all the time?" It made me kind of reevaluate my friendship. Thinking, you've known me for three years, and then you have the nerve to say that. But then I have to keep thinking on an educational level, maybe he doesn't understand fully what it is. (Jason 285 – 289)

Sue does not feel like Tourette syndrome has a major impact on her relationships with colleagues:

I don't think it had any huge impact. I'm trying to think. I'm sure for years a lot of them wondered. But once they found out what it was, then I think if anything, I think after a while they just stopped noticing. And once they knew what it was, it wasn't such a big issue anymore. So I can't say it really changed my relationship with any of them. I mean, I guess sometimes I've always had, and if you know anything about OCD or you have OCD, I've always said that a lot of people with OCD have what I have kind of coined an obsessive sense of justice. Things have to be just. I think that probably at times drove people crazy. If I saw an injustice, I had to right that injustice. That's why I was so involved in teaching and union activities, all kinds of stuff, and I think that probably at times people who just didn't have that probably got annoyed with that. Nobody ever said anything, but once I get on something, it's hard to get me off that path. I don't give up easily. And I can see where that could be annoying to people. But I don't think it really changed my relationships with any of my colleagues at all. (Sue 433 – 444)

Positive Experiences Due to Disclosing at Work

Some participants who disclosed at work had positive experiences due to their disclosure. Many times, people felt like disclosing at work was a strength for them. For some, the feeling of knowledge equals power and the fact that they were educating others about Tourette was a positive experience for them. Michelle feels like she has had some positive experiences at work now that she is open about her Tourette:

> I think so, yes. And I think it's nice when teachers have kids that they are just not really sure about. There's been a few kids over the course of even just working at the building where I'm at, when the kids are little, that the teacher is just not sure. And it's nice with my background, to be able to say, "You know what? It's only one tic. Kids have tics." And just educate teachers that way, that just because they have one tic doesn't mean it's Tourette's syndrome right away. So they're learning in their knowledge too, which I think is really great as educators. (Michelle 320 – 325)

Michelle feels that knowledge is power when it comes to understanding Tourette:

> I don't know if it's a strength so much, but the knowledge again. People can come to me and ask me about their students, or even their own kids. I have another teacher in my school who, her son was just diagnosed in the last year. Just being someone they can come to and someone they can talk to. (Michelle 348 – 351)

Tracey feels like Tourette syndrome is becoming more well-known than it was when she was younger. She also feels like she is in a good profession because education teaches acceptance. She feels that disclosing to her colleagues is a source of strength for her. She feels like she is better equipped to help out with other children with special needs:

> It's showing your colleagues what the children need, maybe their strengths and weaknesses, and helping them get the right information, or showing them where to go for the right information. (Tracey 343 – 345)

Sue believes disclosing at work has given her some strengths she can use on the job:

> It's a double edge sword. In your own building, you're just one of their colleagues, so you're not always.... I went back to my old school a few months ago on behalf of a child with Tourette, and they didn't seem to take me seriously at all. Even though they know that I know a lot about it, I'm just a colleague, a friend. I haven't taught there in a few years, but that's the only place I've ever taught. But I think in other schools, definitely, when I go in, they see me as kind of an expert in the area. Like today, this teacher said to me, "We're getting ready to call the parents in and have a meeting, and I'd like you to come and meet with them, myself, and the school psychologist and the principal. Would you be able to do that?" And she was so thrilled that I would come in and meet with them. She said, "I feel like that as a young teacher, I'm really not understanding what's going on with this kid. And I want to prepare him for next year. And whoever he's going to have, I want him to do well." They really can admit that they don't have a lot of experience in this area, and they don't understand it, and they want to help. And I think in my own district, this was in the district I taught, the school I went to today, they used and abused me all the time. Because they didn't have a lot of knowledge of it,

and they were always calling me in. Another thing is, I know some advocates who will go in and be very judgmental toward teachers, like, "You should know this stuff," and, "How could you be doing this stuff?" And I don't ever do that. Because I know how, as a teacher, that feels. I looked at this teacher today, and she had 22 first graders. I looked at her and I said, "Now I know why I taught middle school." Oh my God! I could never deal with 22 six-year-olds or seven-year-olds or whatever. I look at the job that she has to do in the course of the day and say the same thing over and over, and that one's tattling on this one, and this one and this one. And then this hyperactive child with all his tics on the other side of the room. I give them so much credit. And if we go in and start saying, like today, there were a lot of things she did wrong with this child. There are really a lot of things she did wrong. But she didn't do it on purpose. She's trying, she has a little tally sheet on his desk, she's trying all kinds of strategies, but she just doesn't have the knowledge of this disorder because he was just diagnosed recently. And she hasn't gone to an in-service, I haven't been in to meet with her too much. So I didn't go in and say, "Oh my God, his problem is you." Which, in some ways it was, not totally. But I empathized with her. And I said, "I can see how difficult it is," and I said, "You don't even have a classroom aide, you have 21 other kids." And she said, "So you think this kid needs services?" And I said, "Oh my God, one hundred percent. I wouldn't even bat an eyelash requesting that this child has an IEP." He really, really needs it because one teacher can't do this all. And I think teachers sometimes are afraid to have you come in their classroom because they are so afraid that you're going to blame everything on them.

Sometimes even when you know it's a teacher, I know as a teacher myself, you're not going to get anywhere by walking in the door and blaming the teacher. Even in my own building, I would do that all the time. I would go in and observe classes and watch a child, and even if I felt that it was the teacher causing a lot of the problems, I would never ever say that to them. Because you're done at that point. They resent you. They don't want to listen to anything you have to say. (Sue 759 – 797)

Stacy feels like having Tourette's makes her more willing to stand up for students when the staff seems to be against them. She feels like she will stick up for students that are getting picked on in the faculty lounge.

Challenges Experienced Due to Disclosing at Work

Just as some participants experienced positive outcomes at work because of disclosing, at times, some of them experienced challenges because of disclosing as well. Laura notes that disclosing at work can sometimes bring her challenges:

Sometimes I felt like my colleagues didn't take me as seriously because I'd be blinking or doing whatever. And I felt like they'd be focused on my tics rather than what I was trying to say. (Laura 325 – 326)

She also realizes that people can read her mood by the volume of her tics:

I had a mentor this year, and she could always tell when I was really stressed out because my Tourette's would get worse. Even if I was like, "No, I'm fine," people would be like, "You're not fine.

You're ticcing like crazy." So I guess that makes it harder to put a wall up like that. But I don't know that's really a bad thing. (Laura 332 – 335)

Tracey does not feel like disclosing has presented her with any challenges at work:

> You know, I really don't have any challenges when I work with my colleagues. I think most teachers, and I say most because there are some that just don't, but most teachers really understand. You're not a person with Tourette's or a disability, you're just another colleague and you're a friend. And everybody has their own way, their own teaching style, their own way of doing things, and their own needs and wants. And I feel that teachers sometimes are very understanding to that. I have not had any encounters, but I'm sure that there are older teachers that are set in their ways that would have a hard time understanding. (Tracey 366 – 372)

Just as there are strengths, there are also challenges for Sue with identifying as an educator with Tourette syndrome:

> It wasn't a huge challenge for me. I know there were times when I would run into staff members that were in very set in their ways and in not wanting to believe. And I see this not only in my own school but in a lot of the schools I go to, not wanting to believe that this wasn't something that the child couldn't control. It was much more difficult in my own building because these are colleagues of mine, so it was not like a stranger going into their classroom. It sometimes, I would find myself at odds with the particular teacher because they had a really, really hard time understanding, but to me it was kind of like a challenge. Like, "How can I get to this teacher?"

And, "How can I get them to turn to my way of thinking?" And then I would spend, I'm just obsessive enough to stick on that until I can get this person. So many times, I was able to change their way of thinking. And let them realize… sometimes I have this, when I present, I have a little exercise that I do. It's been published, so you may have seen it somewhere. I make them do a particular writing task, everybody in the audience. And I give them one tic and one obsession. And then I time them. And no one ever finishes. What I have them write is the pledge to the flag, and every time I clap my hands, they have to do one of my tics. One of my most interfering tics that hardly anybody sees is I take my little finger and I hit it on everything. I hit it on the desk when I'm writing, I hit it on the windshield when I'm driving, I'm constantly doing that. So every time I clap my hands, they have to take the little finger of the hand they're writing with and hit it on the page. And every third word, I tell them it doesn't look like it's completely on the line, it doesn't look symmetrical to them, so they have to cross it out and rewrite it so it looks perfect. And I give them a minute and a half, which is plenty of time to do the pledge to the flag without all these interferences. And I give tips to them, and I keep saying, "Don't forget to check your spelling, and watch your neatness; neatness is very important. Don't forget your punctuation, and don't forget.…" Just beating a typical obnoxious teacher. And then I keep clapping my hands and teachers stop in the middle, and they just throw up their hands, and they don't finish. When I finish with them, I'll ask them, "How many of you finished?" And I've never ever, ever had a teacher finish. Ever. I've done this thousands of times. They've never finished. And I'll say to them, "How did you feel when you were doing it?" And then they'll look at me and say, "Horrible. Frustrated. A basket case." And then I'll ask them, "How many quit?" And so many of them will raise their hand. They quit in the middle, and I would go up to them and say, "How do you know you don't know this? You didn't even try. You just stopped in the middle." And I'll say, "Why did you stop?" And they'll all be honest and say because they knew they were never going to finish it. And it was so frustrating. And then I asked them, "How many of you lost track of what you were writing?" And they would say, "The pledge to the flag is one of those things we learn from rote memory, so every time you're interrupted you have to start all over again." And they just completely lost track of what they were doing, and I would say to them, "Did I really give you Tourette? Because I only gave you one tic and one obsession, and Tourette, the first criteria is multiple tics." I'd be shaking my head and jerking my head and clacking my teeth and then hitting my finger; I'd have a million acts going on. And boy, there's nothing more powerful to do to a group of teachers. And to make them really start to understand what these kids are living through. Sometimes I resort to that. I've done that with principals of schools. I had a principal, one time who had been punishing the kid for every little thing, and I had him stand up and read. And every time I clapped my hands, he had to shake his head back and forth. That was one of my tics. And after about maybe a minute, he sat down. And he wouldn't finish. And then he came up to me afterward and then I said, "Are you going to tell me it's a good thing I don't work for you?" And he said, "No, I want to tell you that you really got your point across. I was so humiliated and so embarrassed that I could not read. I could not stand in front of my staff and read because of one tic." So I think sometimes that's what we have to resort to with these teachers. I really feel strongly that it's difficult sometimes for staff members, and it's especially difficult in my own building because they're friends. So how do you get across to them? (Sue 864 – 915)

Discrimination Faced Due to Disclosing

Unfortunately, one participant experienced a situation with discrimination because of having Tourette syndrome. Although Tracey had a situation with a parent of one of her students this year, she still felt supported by her administration:

> Sure, I believe in disclosing that I have Tourette's to my kids, and I actually got that from another teacher with Tourette's syndrome; I went to see him speak and he talked about how he tells his kids and they have a big session about it. So after I listened to him, I said, "Okay, I'm going to see how it works for me." So I started telling my kids, and I've never had a bad reaction. But I had a parent who had a student with a hearing problem, and in the meeting the one day, he had gotten into a fight in the stairwell, just in the middle of the meeting she blurted out how my Tourette's is a disturbance to him and his learning because the noises confuse him, and the arm motions distract from what he's trying to learn. So she wanted him out, this was like halfway through the school year. She said that she'd been trying to get them out of my class, and nobody had heard about it. My principal was very firm with her notion. She told her that my disability has nothing to do with his learning. And that he sits in the front of the classroom, went through all of that.

And she said that the mother could go to whomever she wanted, but until she received something in writing from the superintendent saying that she had to move him, she was not moving him from my classroom. They actually had someone come in and observe me. But they came to observe me, and he was like the perfect student when that person was in there. Which is so funny because he's not like that, but he answered questions, he got them right, he paid attention, he took notes, he was totally a different person. But that was actually a benefit to me because by doing that, he was showing the person observing that he was able to follow along and he was able to understand, and that the Tourette's was not inhibiting him in any way. And she actually put that in the report, that he paid attention, and that he took notes, and that there were no issues. (Tracey 84 – 96, 98 – 105)

She was thankful for the support she received from her administration:

I know I mentioned in the interview last week that I had a student who, the parent felt that my Tourette's was distracting, and I wasn't a good teacher because of that. But, at my workplace, I don't feel like I've had that impact at all. In fact, when the mother wanted a child out of my classroom, my principal was just the opposite. She was like, "No, I'm not going to move her out. That discrimination. She's a wonderful teacher. Why would I do that?" So I really feel, maybe it's because of the teaching profession, I find that teachers are more understanding. (Tracey 231 – 237)

Sue does not feel like she has experienced any discrimination at her workplace because of having Tourette syndrome:

No. I can honestly say at my workplace that's never happened. And I know that it has happened to some people, but I think part of it was my attitude and the fact that they knew me before I got the job because I student taught there, and they'd become accustomed to, even though she has something, we don't know what it is, she seems like she's a stable person and works hard and does a good job, so it became again that overachieving. I became known as that kind of a person. No, I honestly can say I don't think there's ever been a time when I was discriminated against at work. (Sue 514 – 520)

None of the participants ever left a school district because of discrimination experienced at work due to having Tourette syndrome. Sue comments how she stayed at her supportive school district for her entire career:

No. I stayed in the same one for 33 years. I have to say though that I taught in an exceptional school district. It's a suburban school district, and they have always had wonderful services for kids with special needs. That's why a lot of people move into the district. I don't know. Would it have been different in another district? Possibly. Although I had a very close friend who is a Spanish teacher who was blind. She got hired by a suburban school district, and she taught there for 27 years. They made all kinds of accommodations for her, obviously. Somebody had to correct her papers, there was just all kinds of stuff. I think a lot of schools do the right thing, and I really had an exceptional school district. I am blessed that I got the job. (Sue 584 – 591)

Socialization with Colleagues Outside of Work

Many participants socialized at least occasionally with colleagues outside of work. They did not seem to think that having Tourette syndrome hindered their friendships. Laura does socialize with other colleagues outside of school:

> This year, yes I did because I have class every night with 26 other teachers. Two of them were in my building actually. I get together, one of my really good friends works in the district, not at my school, and I met her through school, so we became friends. I don't spend a whole lot of time with people outside of school, but occasionally we'll go shopping together or grab coffee or something. (Laura 200 – 204)

Michelle is friendly with her colleagues and does socialize with them outside of school:

> Occasionally we, maybe once a month or so, a bunch of teachers will get together and go to happy hour type of thing. And that would only be about an hour, hanging out and just talking. (Michelle 226 – 228)

Jason does socialize with colleagues outside of work:

> I ran a lot with colleagues. We go running a lot. I have another good friend that, another colleague, he and I kind of just hung out and watched TV together. (Jason 272 – 273)

Tracey does enjoy socializing with others from work:

> Yeah, we go to happy hour on Fridays, just a bunch of us sitting around chitchatting. There's a girl that I work with that we walk sometimes after school, like a little work out. It's just pretty much your typical

colleagues hanging out, having a good time, chitchatting. (Tracey 187 – 189)

She feels like her Tourette syndrome has not hindered her relationships with colleagues:

I don't think it affects my relationships on a negative note by any means. People are very understanding. I feel like we're all educators, we're all adults so I feel like they're not judging you, and they're very comfortable around me. I get along with everybody, I really do. (Tracey 204 – 206)

Mike also feels comfortable socializing with colleagues outside of work. Many of his teacher friends get together for numerous social events. Sue enjoys socializing outside of work with her colleagues:

I did. I had a lot of, I still have a lot of good friends that are still teaching and some that are retired. And yeah, we had all kinds of activities, we'd go out on a Friday night, a bunch of us would go out, and have, we go out for dinner or whatever. We'd get together on weekends. Yeah, I have a lot of friends who are teachers, and we did stuff. And I was very involved in our teachers union. In my building, I was the senior building rep in our building, and then I went on to be on the executive committee, and I actually did the union newsletter. And so I had a lot of really good friends, and we had a lot of things that we did through that group. I had friends all over the district. Just a lot of different activities. (Sue 395 – 403)

Conclusion

Most of my participants did disclose to some extent while teaching. Some participants waited a little while before they disclosed; they wanted to be viewed as an equal before being viewed as a person with a disability. Many of the participants noted that when they did start disclosing, their colleagues were accepting of them. Participants believed education is integral in others' acceptance of Tourette. It was felt that once people knew about Tourette and understood it, they were extremely accepting of it.

Participants also believed that they were looked at as the resident expert on Tourette syndrome. Administrators called on them to assist with students in the district who had Tourette. Other than asking for assistance, administrators did not seem fazed by the fact that one of their employees had Tourette syndrome. Educators with Tourette felt proud that their administrators called on them for assistance in other situations in the district.

Some of the participants stated their Tourette was less stressful after they had disclosed. Symptoms worsen when one is anxious, but when the pressure to suppress one's tics has been alleviated, a person is not as anxious. When you are consciously trying to suppress your tics, it is harder to do so. One participant noted that after her colleagues knew she had Tourette, she wasn't worried if she ticced in front of them.

Colleagues, as well as administrators, were supportive after participants disclosed. Participants stated that they needed to be open, honest, and comfortable when discussing Tourette with others. Many participants felt positive that they were educating others about Tourette. One commented that she truly believed she was viewed as a colleague and a friend, and not as a person with a disability. Many participants socialized with colleagues outside of work and did not think that Tourette syndrome hindered their friendships. For all of my participants who did disclose at work, they felt that this was a positive experience for them.

CHAPTER SIX

DISCLOSING TO STUDENTS

Purpose

In this chapter, I will examine the common themes found in participants' decisions on whether or not to disclose to students and their parents. In this chapter, I focused on six specific questions: 1) How do you disclose to your students once you are working? 2) How does Tourette syndrome impact your relationships with your students? 3) How do you answer questions about Tourette syndrome? 4) What strengths does identifying as an educator with Tourette syndrome give you? 5) What challenges does identifying as an educator with Tourette syndrome give you? 6) In what ways has disclosing at school empowered you? In answering these questions, I found ten common themes related to disclosing to students. They are: 1) disclosing to students, 2) students' reactions, 3) the impact Tourette syndrome has on relationships with students, 4) disclosing to parents, 5) answering questions about Tourette syndrome, 6) strengths when working with students, 7) strengths when working with families, 8) challenges due to disclosing, 9) empowerment in disclosing, 10) and understanding for students with special needs. I will explore these themes in detail in this chapter.

Disclosing to Students

When Laura started her first year teaching, she was not sure what she would say to her students. She decided to say nothing and see how it played out. Students did start to notice and ask questions, so she was honest with them:

It does affect me daily, so my students did notice. And they kept asking me, "Are you okay? Why do you keep blinking so much? You're making funny noises." And so I guess about the third week of school, I sat them down, and I told them, I said, "I have this thing called Tourette's syndrome." I read them a picture book called *Tic Talk*. It's written from the perspective of, it's like a nine-year-old boy who has Tourette's, and it's a true story. But it's written in kid language, so it really helped them. And from then on out, my students and I, we were really open about it. They would sometimes be like, "Oh, is your Tourette's bad today?" And I would say, "Yeah, it is a little bad, but that's okay." They could just tell. They actually started to gauge my mood by it. They would say, "You're tired today, aren't you?" I would say, "Why do you say that?" They would say, "You're blinking a lot." So it became really open. And we actually had an Abilities Awareness Day for fifth graders, and I presented on Tourette's. And it was really cool to be able to share with the kids about this disorder that is so stigmatized as shouting out cuss words, when really that's coprolalia, which is such a subset of the Tourette's population. And I don't have coprolalia, thank goodness. But just to educate them. And they are so accepting of it. And they're going to grow up to be accepting adults then. So that was really cool. (Laura 58 – 73)

Michelle just started disclosing to her students the past few years:

My students are starting to know now because with my kids having it, and teachers are asking me about it all the time, so my students are hearing about it. With James Durbin that was just on *American Idol*, I had his picture from our local newspaper, I had that hanging in my room, so when kids would ask, if they asked about it, I would tell them, "Well my kids have it, and I have it." So the students are starting to know more, so that's kind of new for me because they've not known up until just the last couple of years. (Michelle 26 – 31)

She has been the most open about disclosing this year:

Yes, and honestly, I guess what started it was the whole *American Idol* thing. I've always kind of liked *Idol*, I've never bothered to vote for anybody, never cared that much. My kids watch it; we've never voted. And this year, I guess, first of all, James Durbin having Tourette's is an awesome thing because lots of kids got to see it, but in addition, he was really good. So we really thought he was just really good. So I started to vote for him and then like I said, there was the article in the paper with his picture and then a picture with a younger kid who had Tourette's who looks up to him. So someone had given me the article, one of the teachers, so I hung it up in my room. And then as I said, kids would ask, "Why do you have James Durbin on the wall? What's that about?" And I would always start off with, "Well, you know how he makes funny faces and things like that when they're talking to him?" I said, "He has Tourette's syndrome." It was surprising that a lot of the kids didn't know. They knew he made the faces on TV, but they missed the part that he had Tourette's and that he couldn't help doing that. So we talked about it. We took it as a moment where I could teach them a little bit about that, and then I would go on to say that both my kids have it. My kids' pictures were there so that we would talk about that. And then I told them, "That's what I have." And they would say, "You don't do that. You don't make faces. You don't do any of that." Then I feel kind of bad because I'm telling them, "Well, you're right, I don't, but that's because I control it, but you shouldn't control it." So it's kind of like this weird, for nine years I've been telling my kids, don't control it. You just have to tic, but at the same time, that's what I do. I hold it in all the time. So that's kind of a weird thing. It's been kind of neat. Because as different kids come into the room, I had this after school class. I told the after school kids because they were talking about the picture, but then some of those kids came to my speech class too. So the one who made the comment, "Oh, he is that really weird guy that make those faces." So we talked all about it and why does he do it and all this sort of stuff. And then when that same kid came to speech class later with four different kids, he started telling those kids, "That's the guy from *American Idol* and he has this thing. Oh, what's it called again, Mrs. Browning?" And so here he was three days before saying, "Oh, that's that weird guy that makes faces," and now there he is teaching the other kids and telling the other kids, "Oh, Mrs. Browning does that and her kids do that, and they can't help it." It was kind of cool. (Michelle 114 – 141)

At this point in Jason's career, he has only told a few students about having Tourette syndrome. Therefore, Jason does not consider himself to be someone who discloses to the students:

And I don't even tell students. I just did that with the one student because he did, because he had it, and I knew he had it. And the parent at that time was in denial as well. Because she thought the same thing, well, he doesn't cuss and whatever. I talked to her about it and gave her some books and some videos about it. Every year I show that video from

HBO *I Have Tourette's but Tourette's Doesn't Have Me*. I show that video to the class. And I tell them what Tourette's is. None of them have ever asked why I show it, I just say, "We're going to learn about a disability today. I want you guys to know about it." (Jason 135 – 144)

Tracey discloses to her students at the start of every school year:

They ask questions. They're genuinely concerned, kind of confused, "Well, what do you mean?" and I have to show them, "Listen, I do these arm movements and I do this, and I make these noises." And then we talk about how there's other kids in our class and in the school who have disabilities, whether it's ADHD or whether they're smaller than everybody else or taller than everybody. Everybody has a disability, and we don't want to make fun of those children, we have to be understanding. And the kids are very understanding. Every now and then I'll have a kid, you know I might do something different and they'll go, "Mrs. Miller, is that a new tic?" And I laugh and I'm like, "Yeah, it is." But I remember, when I taught fifth grade, I had this boy and he had a lazy eye. One of the kids laughed at him. And one of the girls said to him, "Don't laugh at him. That's like laughing at Mrs. Miller. You wouldn't laugh at Mrs. Miller, would you?" And the little boy stopped, and he apologized. So you don't realize the impact it has on them. It was just amazing how this little girl was like, "That's like laughing at Mrs. Miller. You wouldn't do that." And the little boy stopped. It never occurred to him because we had talked about my disability, but he had never related it to other children. So it's nice to see their acceptance with how they are with other children. Just because of this disability, we're able to talk about acceptance of other children. It really is wonderful. (Tracey 107 – 122)

Mike discloses to his students the first day of every school year:

And we sat down on the first day, and we educated all the kids. I knew that if I educated the kids, they would go home and educate their parents. And that's what I did. I educated them, and they went home, and parents had, they had some reservations about this. But they realized if their kid didn't have a problem, then they didn't. Quickly, we formed those relationships, and the student learning started to happen, and I was able to be myself, and they were able to be themselves. And after a year, we had a lot of big successes. I definitely did not have an easy class my first year; there were a lot of challenges. But I let the students know that I wouldn't give up on them because I knew what it was like for someone to give up on me. And I stayed with them late. We practiced reading and math and writing. We worked on all of our issues. And I'm not saying that I was perfect, but I gave everything I could. And I feel like I was a better teacher because of some of the negative and positive experiences that I had had in life. My goal was to make sure that other kids didn't have to go through what I went through. I was honored that after my first year of teaching, I was elected as the First Class Teacher of the Year from our state. I really had the opportunity to be that role model for the kids. That just one year prior to getting my job, I had principals saying that I couldn't do it, and now after my first year of teaching, I'm been recognized by the entire state for what I was able to do. Not that that award means everything and that I'm the best teacher, but I think what it did say is that,

"Hey, you're making a difference." I think that having that acknowledgement really helped me. And so for 15 years I've been an educator and by getting that first award, I think it helped me to remember to keep high expectations for my students and myself and to make a difference. I know that people's eyes are always on me and many times, they're waiting for me to mess up because I have Tourette's syndrome. I never allowed them to even get to the point to think that Tourette's is going to be a hindrance because I tried to show off all my other strengths. And that's what I tried to do with my students too. So I've been educating, and I still have Tourette's. It's part of who I am. Some people say it goes away as you get older, I'm still waiting to get older I guess. The tics are still around. I have vocal tics; I have facial tics. I do what I do, and I've pretty much had it for my whole life. And that's who I am. (Mike 80 – 106)

As soon as Sue was diagnosed, she started disclosing to her students. In fact, she would even discuss her tics with students before she had a name for it:

You know, the first few days of school, I would always tell my students, just so they knew. Because before that, they would look at me, and they would ask me why I was doing those things; they would keep track on paper how many times I was doing things, and I had no response to them. It was very upsetting, but I had no response. And now I can tell them something. And, I see those students all the time. I was in a school this morning doing a little workshop on behalf of a student with Tourette, and one of the teachers in that school was one of my former students. And that happens to me all the time. She came up and hugged me and said, "Oh my God, you must have been so relieved. I remember you doing all those things, but," she said, "After a while, you were just you. And we didn't even notice it anymore." And that made me feel good because I was always so self-conscious. But that's life. You've kind of have to plug ahead with things. I'm not going to stay home and hide because I have Tourette. That's just always been my attitude. (Sue 150 – 162)

Stacy does not disclose to her students.

Students' Reactions

Laura believed her students were very supportive:

They took it really well. I kind of took the approach that we're all different, and we all have our own struggles. This is just something that I have to deal with. I was born with it. And I can't change it. It's just like I have blonde hair and maybe you have brown hair or black hair. It's just how I was born, and that's just who I am. And they were really fine with it. They never made fun of it. And I actually, it was kind of fun, I heard them educating other students on it. I used the phrase, "It's like a hiccup in your brain." And I heard them telling other kids that, "My teacher has Tourette's. It's like hiccups in your brain." And they learn from it. (Laura 119 – 125)

She thinks kids, by nature, are adaptive and accepting. She also knows that education is the key. Once you educate them about Tourette syndrome, they are fine with it:

Yeah, and my librarian was someone that I shared it with before the school year started. She was like, "I'll use part of the library budget to get some books on Tourette's." And so she did, and so the kids were able to go and check them out and read them, and it was good. (Laura 128 – 131)

Michelle's students took the news very well:

> They just had lots of questions. I answered their questions. Especially young kids, when you answer their questions and they have the information, they're just kind of cool with it. (Michelle 163 – 164)

She thinks that kids are very adaptive:

> I don't know about middle school or high school, how that would be, but at the elementary level, it didn't faze them. They asked their questions and then we moved on. (Michelle 166 – 167)

When Jason has disclosed to students in the past, he reflects on how they took the news:

> I don't tell many. Like I said, I'll just tell the ones who like the kid who had Tourette's, I talked to him. Because he was having issues at the time with kids, not only the sub, but a couple kids were starting to mimic him. His was a lot worse than mine. They were mimicking him a lot because he did a lot of noises, and he used to do it out loud in class. He had no control. And so I talked to him a little bit. He was kind of embarrassed even with me talking about it. And I kept telling him, "Man, I've lived with this. I've had teachers mimic me in the past." I said, "I know what you're going through." I said, "Education. You just got educate people about this stuff. That's what you have to do. And if they don't know what it is, they're going to make fun of it." I said, "That's just a fact. It's human nature. If someone's uncomfortable with something, they're

just going to, probably, make a joke of it, unless they know what it is." I said, "You just can't let people not know what you have." I think he got a little bit better with it. But as far as other students, some kids don't quite understand it. But when I showed the video to all the other kids when I talked about Tourette's, not that I had it, but when I talked about it, they all seem to say, "Oh that's sad that these kids have to live with that." And I said, "But guys, keep in mind, these kids are just normal, just like you, they just have different little quirks about them." And they all seemed fine with it though. (Jason 186 – 201)

Mike's students adapt to Tourette extremely well:

I gave them a question and answer period. They asked me lots of questions. I'd say the first five, six, seven questions were geared towards me and Tourette's syndrome. And then after that, they just wanted to get to know me as a person. It kind of makes you chuckle that it didn't take them long to look past the Tourette's. (Mike 132 – 135)

Sue's students dealt with the information very well:

They were fine with it. I wouldn't say anything until somebody brought it up. And that usually happened the first day. Because, middle school students in particular, they can be not so kind. As you know, it's not the kindest age on Earth. I'd see somebody in the back keeping track of how many times I did each tic, and then I would say, "You probably wonder why I'm doing these things." And I would just open up and tell them what it was. And once I told them, then that was, I was very open about it, that was the end of the issue. And I would say to them, "I'm willing to bet, within a couple of days, you won't even notice it anymore because you're just going to get used to it. And that's the way it is." And they did. And they tell me that today when I see them. "After a while that was just you; we never noticed it anymore." That was the good news. (Sue 207 – 216)

Sue never had any negative situations with students or parents because of having Tourette syndrome:

I mean, I know that people probably wondered and people probably said things, but again, I was always one of those people who had to be an overachiever. I had to, I did millions of things with the kids. I was running field trips; I ran Student Council; I did French club. I was very active, and so I think it just made me a more valuable teacher to them. I was determined, "You're not going to get rid of me because of this." (Sue 226 – 230)

Impact Tourette Syndrome Has on Relationships with Students

Laura believed her Tourette had a positive impact on her relationships with her students:

I think it was a positive impact on my relationship with students because they saw that I struggled with something as well. I think it really helped them relate, like when they were frustrated with things. I had one little girl who was frustrated with her ADHD or frustrated with certain things, and I was like, "You know what, I get it. I get frustrated too. I get angry that I have to deal with Tourette's." I think it was good for them to see that I was still able to do what I want as an adult. I was still able to

156

become a teacher and overcome that and not let it
define me. (Laura 220 – 225)

Michelle does not feel like her Tourette impacts her
relationships with her students:

> I don't think my Tourette's really does impact it. It's
> really not bad. It's not a severe case. So it really
> doesn't affect that. They might ask questions, I
> answer them, and that's pretty much it. (Michelle
> 248 – 249)

Tracey feels like her Tourette syndrome has a positive
impact on her relationship with her students:

> It's kind of like I said before. First of all, I think it's
> a very good impact because I find that I'm very
> understanding with the kids. I had a little girl in my
> class this year, believe it or not, she had Tourette's
> syndrome. And it was very different, but I
> understood when she was unorganized and her dad
> would be calling, "She forgot her book." At the end
> of the day, "Amy, let me check your book bag, let
> me make sure you have this." I really felt for her,
> and I feel for the kids that have the ADHD or a
> student that is not attentive because you've been
> through that and you understand sometimes they
> can't control it. So I feel like it has a good impact.
> And I feel like they're at such a young age where
> they're not at the age quite yet where they can start
> ridiculing you and seeing the negative aspects of it.
> For them it's like, "Oh, Mrs. Miller has something,
> you know she just has a problem," but they learn to
> deal with it. (Tracey 208 – 217)

Sue does not think Tourette syndrome impacted her
relationship with students at all:

No. It really didn't. I mean, they would say things that, the 15 years I taught before I knew what it was, they would ask about it. I would just say, "I don't know. I've had this for years. I'm not sure what it is. I've gone to a lot of doctors. Nobody seems to know." I actually had a couple of things I used to do. At the beginning of the year, before I knew I had Tourette, I would watch the kids kind of keeping track in the back of the room those first couple days, the times I did a certain tic. And I developed these couple of strategies that actually did work quite well. One of them was to go back to where the kid was keeping track and say, "I think you forgot one." They would get very nervous about that. And my favorite thing to do was to speed up my tics. So that they were so fast they couldn't keep up with it. And they just stopped doing it because they figured, whatever, there's no sense in trying to do this, she's doing it so fast. Once I knew what it was, and they asked me about it, I'd just tell them. And kids are amazingly understanding and forgiving if they just know what it is. And I just didn't let it be anything that was going to change me as a teacher. This is me. This is what I do. And I used to say to them, "Everybody's different. Look around the room. I don't have two people in this room that are exactly the same. Everybody has something, and this is just what I have." I'd explain what it was, and that would be the end of it. I'd never hear about it again. I don't think I really did. I think if anything, as I said before, it definitely made me a much more empathetic, understanding teacher. But I don't think it changed my relationship with my students at all. (Sue 446 – 463)

Disclosing to Parents

Laura decided to tell the parents of her students on a need-to-know basis:

> I didn't tell parents straight out. I had one set of parents that I did tell because their child struggles with OCD and anxiety as well. And she was having a hard time with the diagnosis and having to go to counseling. And I kind of pulled her aside and I was talking to her parents, and I said, "I did this too." I just kind of talked about it. And so the parents I was closer to figured it out. The ones that came and picked their kids up every day. They knew, just from seeing me. But it never really was a huge issue. (Laura 133 – 138)

She understood that many of her kids would go home and educate their parents after she educated them.

Tracey discloses to parents as well:

> I have never had any parent react negatively. I put it in the newsletter when I go through and I tell them I do have Tourette's syndrome, and I actually have parents that are very happy, especially if they have children with a disability. I had one mother who said she liked the fact that I have a disability because it made me more receptive and understanding and sympathetic to her child that had disabilities. The impression I get from them is they feel it makes me a better teacher because I am so easy-going and nurturing. (Tracey 124 – 129)

Mike talks about the parents reacting to the news:

> At first, there was a lot of reservation. But then, I think they saw that once that they noticed that their kid didn't have a problem with it, then they didn't

need to either. Definitely, there was some reservation. There was one or two that had a problem with it. The administration said to me, "Mike, we're going to move this student from your class." And I was upset. I was like, "What are you talking about?" And they moved the kid from my class, just because they realized, you know what, this is a high maintenance parent, always has been. I might have not understood everything at that time, but they could see the bigger picture. They decided to move the kid from my class. The ironic thing is, three weeks later, that same parent realized that they made a mistake, and they asked that their child be moved back into my class. And the administrator said, "No, too late." (Mike 137 – 145)

Answering Questions About Tourette Syndrome

Laura answers questions about Tourette syndrome openly and honestly. Michelle feels it is important to be honest when answering their questions about Tourette. She discusses how she answers their questions:

As honestly as I possibly can. And at the same time, they're kids. Their understanding is more limited than adults, so it's pretty simple in terms of the language that I use. Sue, who is a good friend, as you know, I've listened to her explain it to young kids when she was going into my daughter's classes and explaining it. So, I kind of took from what she had said if kids have questions like, "Can you catch it? Does everybody in the family have it?" Kids are more familiar with things like asthma and diabetes. So compared to that type of thing, you wouldn't make fun of a kid who has diabetes, you wouldn't make fun of a kid who has asthma. They can't help

160

it; it's just the way that their body was made type of thing. So I've taken what I've seen Sue say to kids. And just do my best to be honest about it. (Michelle 251 – 259)

Jason answers questions about Tourette:

I just answer it based on how it's affected me or what I've read. I tried to just educate people and tell them what I know about it. If they don't know, I'll try to tell them. (Jason 291 – 292)

He believes education is imperative in Tourette syndrome becoming accepted by everyone:

Yes. I found that out with that sub. She had no idea what it was, and she was giving a kid a hard time. And that's why I tried to tell the mother, "She doesn't know what it is." And the mother was like, "Well, she's a sub in this corporation, and she should know better. She should have some sense." Yes, she should have some sense, but it's also a sub trying to get a study hall room at a middle school level calmed down, and if the kid's making noises, she may not have thought through that process. (Jason 294 – 299)

Tracey answers questions about Tourette honestly:

I tried to answer it as honest as I can. When they ask a question about it, I tell them that it's something I was born with. I show them some of the facial tics and the arm tics that I may do. I tell them that at any time if they have any questions or if my tics confuse them, they can come up and talk to me. But with the kids, I am very honest about it. I find with adults, it's a little harder to be honest about it. I mean they know that there's something wrong, but it's hard to be like, "Oh, I have

Tourette's syndrome, and I do this, this, and this."
But I feel like the kids might see some of your
quirks a little more than adults might. (Tracey 222
– 228)

Mike answers questions about Tourette honestly:

I am open and honest. I always look at it as an
opportunity to educate other people. If I can educate
more people, that makes it easier for people who
have Tourette's now, then mission accomplished.
(Mike 228 – 230)

Sue answers questions about Tourette honestly:

I'm usually very direct. Very direct. If someone
looks at me, I try to hit it off. You know I travel a
lot, I do presentations, and if I'm on an airplane, and
I keep seeing someone kind of looking over at me,
I'll say, "I'm sorry, I have Tourette syndrome. Do
you know what that is?" And very often, you get
into this great discussion. It's very interesting. I was
on a plane going out to the West Coast to do a
program, and I think I was in Washington, in the
state of Washington, and there was a family, a man
sitting next to me, and he asked me about it, and I
told him. And we started talking about it, and he
said, "You're not going to believe this, but my
fiancé has a son, and he's eight years old, and he
was just diagnosed with this." He said, "As a matter
of fact, I'm going out to the West Coast now to
visit. They live in the state of Washington." And I
told him about the seminar that I was presenting,
and when I got to the seminar the next afternoon, he
and his fiancée were there. It was so neat. He was
so excited that somebody was going to talk about
Tourette, and he said, "She really needs to hear this.
I really need to hear this. I don't understand her

son," and they came, and they spent the afternoon, and I've heard from them several times since. I think if you're direct about it and just tell people what it is. Are you going to run into people who don't understand, yes. I've had that happen. I've had it happen on planes, in movie theaters. I was in a movie theater one time; this lady came over. I had positioned myself, it was a weekday afternoon, so there were about maybe nine people in the theater, so I positioned myself way over to the side so that people wouldn't be near me, and she came over and sat right in back of me. And I turned around, and I said, "I'm just going to warn you that I have Tourette syndrome, and that's why I'm sitting way over here on the side. So, just so you know." The movie started, and she immediately started complaining. And she actually went out and got the usher and brought the usher in. And I wanted to say, "You know, I gave her fair warning." But instead I moved to somewhere else in the theater. Finally, I decided I was just going to leave because that whole thing stressed me out, which made the tics worse. I wasn't enjoying myself. You know, I went to the movie to see a movie and enjoy myself, but when you're worried about other people saying things, I just wasn't enjoying myself. And you're going to meet those people everywhere. People who just don't think you can't stop doing that, and they make these comments, but I think if you're very open and very direct with them, it's usually the best way to handle it. (Sue 465 – 493)

Strengths When Working with Students

Laura also feels like identifying as an educator with Tourette syndrome is a strength when working with students:

> I think students can relate to the fact that I have struggles too. And I think it helps them to accept the fact that everyone's different. I can tell them some days, "Hey, I'm struggling with my Tourette's. I understand that you're frustrated with whatever you're doing. I get frustrated too." I think it just helps them understand that it's normal to be frustrated and to have to deal with things. (Laura 289 – 293)

She also feels that disclosing to her students gave way to some positive experiences at her workplace:

> Oh, for sure. One of them is I got to speak at Ability Awareness Day. It was really good to be able to share my story with the kids. And some of the other teachers were in there and the counselor, and they were able to hear more about it and what it's like and really learn about it. I bonded with my librarian over it because she helped me pick out books to order for the school. And she was just really understanding the whole time, and I don't think we would've, I don't think I would've initiated that relationship had we not had that to base it on. (Laura 251 – 256)

Michelle believes that identifying as an educator with Tourette syndrome gives her some strengths when working with students:

> I think acceptance, for one. And I think that true understanding, especially of the related disorders. I think you have a real hands-on feel for all of that. Especially in my position where I work with so

many kids in the building, and even being on the child study team, that I don't necessarily work with the kid, but just to have that background and be able to share that with everyone. So the knowledge base I think is a big strength. (Michelle 332 – 336)

Jason has had some positive experiences at work from disclosing that he has Tourette syndrome:

I think, just getting to educate the staff and even the kids who don't know that I have it, getting to educate them on what it is, subliminally. Not telling them that I have it but just showing them the video and talking about Tourette's. My first year I showed that HBO special to my first group of kids, but the second year I showed that same video, and they liked it so well, I ended up showing *Front of the Class*, the Hallmark show. I showed that also to the kids, and they really liked that. And those kids had a really good sense of what it was, I thought. This is just based off the two videos, but by that and discussing what it was, I think the best thing that I got out of it was that I've educated, what, 500 plus kids in three years on what Tourette's is. So if they come across it, like that one girl telling that teacher, "Hey that teacher down there is giving so-and-so a hard time; I think he has Tourette's." That kid would've never known that, had I not shown that video. So I think that's a pretty good positive experience for me. (Jason 308 – 318)

He believes one strength in being an educator with Tourette syndrome and working with students is communication:

I think communication is probably a strength that it gives me. Just like with that boy, and the fact that no one knew, just keeping an open sense of communication with parents and everybody else. It has just taught me that everybody needs to know everything. If I keep hiding behind not telling people, and then kids are wondering why Mr. Marks does weird things, I think that would be a problem for me. So I think I need to communicate better about that. (Jason 342 – 346)

Mike has had some positive experiences at work because of having Tourette syndrome:

Other kids with Tourette's have transferred to my school because their parents thought they would have a positive role model in their life. That's definitely a humbling experience. So that is definitely a nice thing. Beyond that, it's just again, being a role model and showing the kids with special needs—there's so many kids with special needs, and they just need to know that they don't have to let the challenges get in the way of fulfilling their dreams. (Mike 246 – 251)

Mike also believes there are strengths in being an educator with Tourette syndrome:

For me, I don't think that I'd be the teacher that I am if I didn't go through some of the experiences that I did. I have a friend that was a straight-A student her whole life. She never got a B. And she became a teacher, and one day at work, she was working with a student that struggled so much, and I remember having a conversation with her. And she couldn't get it. She couldn't understand what the issue was with this girl. Through conversation, it eventually came out that she had never struggled herself. So, if you never struggled yourself, you never know what it's like to be in that situation. I'm not saying that she can't help that kid, but I think it's going to be a little more challenging than it would be for someone like me. For me, I know what it's like for somebody to give up on me; I know what it was like for someone not to believe in me; I know what it was like to struggle just to read or to learn to read because I had trouble doing it because of my own issue. But I think that when I see other students struggling for some reason, I can relate to them because I have been there before. Not only can I help them, but I can be that role model and can say, "Hey, I was in your shoes. But I'm not going to give up on you, number one, and number two, we're going to figure this out, and you're going to learn it." I think there's something in that that is very reassuring for those students. And I think that's what I'm able to bring to my classroom. I'm able to bring that approach and that whole mindset that you don't have to treat all kids equal, and everyone doesn't have to be the same. I'll say to someone, "If that kid doesn't get it, have you thought about allowing that kid to only do 10 problems while the rest of the class does all 30?" And they respond, "No, that's not fair. We can't do that." And then I say, "Why not?" If this kid already knows it, and this kid doesn't and struggles, why would you make them do the same thing? That doesn't make sense. Sometimes it's hard for people to get that. We usually hear things like, "Well, if this parent hears that this parent has a kid that only has to do this, but this kid has to do this, they're not going to be happy." You've got to think differently. And so I think that I bring that mindset to my classroom. (Mike 257 – 280)

Sue has had many positive experiences at her workplace due to having Tourette:

A lot of things with the kids. Kids will come up and say, "You are so brave. I don't know that I'd be able to tell people. You make me really think about sharing some of the things that I have." What also happened is that in my district, I became kind of the go-to person if we had anybody else in the district. When I retired, I came from a big school district, when I retired, there were about 43 kids in the district that had Tourette. And they would constantly cover my classes, so I could go over to another building and counsel with the teachers and work with them and do a little in-service. My district has brought me in many, many times for staff development day programs to educate the other teachers all over the district. So they started really, as I always said, using and abusing me. But that was a positive thing; it's taking a negative thing and turning it into a positive. And so they respected me for the information that I had to share with them, and in the long-run, it helped them learn how to deal with these kids. And even now that I'm retired, as a matter of fact, I looked at my calendar sitting next to me, I have three, within the next week, I have three visits back to my school district I taught in to meet with teachers. One is an IEP meeting, and the other two are just little in-service programs that I'm doing. They call me all the time. Actually one of them is to observe a second grader just because they want me to see the kind of struggles he's having so that I can kind of advise them what accommodations they can put in place for this child. And so they've turned it into a positive. Which I think is great. (Sue 552 – 539)

She's had many positive experiences in the classroom:

There were so many. It happened on quite a regular basis. I know I got very involved for a long time, and still do occasionally, with the media. I was able to be on several national television programs. At first I was a little nervous, being a teacher and doing this, but I thought, "I was diagnosed through a television program, so why should I be reluctant to go on a television program?" So I did. And I think I'd rather see someone like myself who is at least a good spokesperson for the disorder rather than other people who probably wouldn't be such a good spokesperson because I wouldn't focus on the sensationalist part of it, and I have a more positive slant on it, and I think that's what we want the media to see. So the kids often see me on television, and they were always extremely complementary. When I would come back, they would want to see all the pictures. At one time I had to go out, I went out to Hollywood actually, and I received an award, a lifetime achievement award, and it was presented to me by Richard Dreyfuss, whom I've always adored. And it was an audience of celebrities. I met so many people there. And of course, when I came back, we had a whole class to look at the pictures of all the celebrities I had met. And they were just so excited. I was taking a negative and turning it into a positive. So many kids would say that to me. In particular, kids with special needs. Because they realized how embarrassed they were by what their difficulty was, whether it be ADHD or a learning disability or a seizure disorder, whatever. And kids would tell me all the time, "You give me the courage to face what I have to face because you just do it, and you don't let it stop you from doing whatever you want to do." I constantly got those kinds of comments from students, and to me, that's what it's all about. That's what I want them to take away from this. That's the message I want them to take away. That it's all right to be different, and it's all right to have a disability, it doesn't make you less of a person. And you've got to get out there and let people understand what's wrong and what's going on, and then people will understand. (Sue 542 – 564)

Having Tourette syndrome did not make it difficult for Sue in leading extracurricular activities:

In school, no. Not really. I ran a lot of the extracurricular activities. I had a very active French club; I took students to France every year for 25 years. I think it was something that I wanted to do. I guess I decided early on whatever this is, it's not going to stop me. I have dreams, and this is what I want to accomplish in life and go for it. You can do what you want to do. That attitude is something that I want everybody else, all the kids that I work with, to have also. I think the best way to teach kids is by role modeling. (Sue 577 – 582)

Sue believes there are strengths in identifying as an educator with Tourette syndrome when working with students:

As I said before, I think the strengths are probably empathy and understanding of kids with any kind of special needs. When you've lived with these kind of problems and issues yourself and been misjudged, mistreated, misunderstood, and all those things, I think you realize, we always say, "Don't judge a book by its cover," and it couldn't be more true with kids with these disorders. I'm sure you've heard of Ross Greene and the guy who wrote the book *The Explosive Child*, and he talks about, one of my favorite quotes of his is, "It's your explanation of the behavior that leads directly to how you respond to it." And then as teachers, we judge kids by certain behaviors, and I think, as a person with Tourette, I came very quickly to realize just because it looks like this doesn't necessarily mean that is who the kid was. And to me, that is a huge strength. I was in the classroom this morning, a first grade class, I had been consulted to come in and observe this child. And the teacher really is a very good teacher. She knows he has Tourette, she knows he has ADHD, and she said to me something. And I met with her before, and halfway through the class, she came back and spoke to me and said, "Do you see how attention seeking he is?" And I kind of looked at her like, "Attention seeking? I don't see one thing about this child that is attention seeking." But in her eyes, as a person who doesn't understand kids with these kind of disorders, his hyperactivity, his inability to sit still in his chair, his very, very complex tics and standing up and doing a little leaping movement, and he's got some real complex hand and neck tics and finger tics, and to her, that was attention seeking. I guess from somebody who doesn't understand these disorders, yeah. So when you think of a kid as attention seeking, you have a totally different explanation and image of this child than if you think this is just part of his neurological disorder, he can't help it. He's not doing that, obviously, he doesn't want to get this kind of negative attention. I think that's, for someone with Tourette, and who can teach, I think that's one of the strengths. You do understand kids who aren't all, I would always say, "Just because it quacks doesn't mean it's a duck. It could be a kid with a quacking tic." I think that's one of the things that was a real strength of mine is being able to see kids for who they are and not necessarily what they appear to be. And also I think it was very helpful to understand kids' learning differences. When you're working with kids, not everybody learns the same way. Sometimes you just have to, I know a lot of teachers that I worked with over the years, when the kids would all fail a test, they'd be in the faculty room correcting papers saying, "Oh my God, I went over this so many times and obviously these kids didn't study." And my reaction if everybody was failing my tests was, "What did I do wrong? Why is everybody failing this test? I obviously didn't teach this very well." And I realized that there was probably learning differences I hadn't taken into consideration. I think those are probably the strengths of a person teaching with Tourette. The other thing I think I realized, and I saw this a lot, also with another teacher with Tourette syndrome, is that kids with attention problems need to be constantly stimulated to pay attention. If you don't grab their attention, kids are not necessarily passive learners. They need to be directly involved in doing things to be able to learn, and I think that's something that a lot of teachers forget about. They lecture, lecture, lecture. And the kids sit there for hours on end. Some kids will do okay with that, but the vast majority of kids just don't learn that way, especially younger kids. They're more active learners, so they've got to at some point be participating in the whole process actively. I think there are a lot of strengths you get from growing up with a disorder like this and then going into a classroom to teach kids. (Sue 673 – 715)

Stacy does feel like there is a strength in having Tourette and working with students:

I think I am more understanding of people and more supportive of kids who are a little bit different or have some kind of issue that they don't have control over. I can support them based on that. (Stacy 151 – 152)

Strengths When Working with Families

Similarly, Laura feels being an educator with Tourette syndrome can be a strength when working with families of students as well:

> I have found experiences here where it really helped me grow in a relationship with the family because they were going through their daughter being diagnosed with some OCD and different things, wondering about different medications. And they came to me quite a bit, actually and asked me what I thought because I've been through it and how it affected my education. Just different things like that. (Laura 296 – 300)

Similarly, Michelle feels like there are strengths in being an educator with Tourette syndrome when working with families as well:

> I think it gives me a real understanding. Especially being the disorganized teacher, the executive functioning difficulties. I think it's nice to be able to share with parents that I have some of the same difficulties, and I use my obsessive compulsiveness to help me along the way. Kind of let them know that you can get through it anyway. On top of that, I have my own kids with it, so oftentimes as a speech therapist, I am the first link in getting kids to the special education realm of education. So I think it's very helpful to be able to say, "I get how hard it is. I understand it. Don't be afraid. It's going to be okay." So I think that helps a lot. (Michelle 339 – 345)

Tracey has had some positive experiences with students due to having Tourette:

I had a girl when I was in fifth grade, and her mother just really loved her in my class. And the mother felt that any time there was an issue, we were able to talk about it, and she felt, I remember her telling me she felt that I gave her child the best care ever because of my disability. I was able to relate to hers. And I really feel like, I don't know, I just keep coming back to that. But as a teacher, I feel like because you have a disability, you can relate to children more with a disability. And I feel like on a positive note, we are able to talk about how everyone, whether you have diabetes or ADHD or any kind of disability, we need understanding and acceptance in regards to that. So I really feel that it has been a blessing in helping to teach. (Tracey 258 – 265)

Tracey believes there are strengths to being an educator with Tourette syndrome and working with students:

The strengths it gives me are I think patience and understanding to other children with disabilities and just to children in general. Not rushing them and understanding for all of them. (Tracey 229 – 230)

She also believes there are strengths when working with families:

With education, working with families, I think it helps parents, I think to be understanding with parents, and I think parents can learn a lot from teachers. You always hear from parents when they talk about how it's easier to hire a tutor than it is for them to work with their own children. And I think a lot of times especially growing up with it, we may know more about Tourette's than parents themselves do. And we can show them where to get the right materials and how to work with their children and how to be more patient and understanding. And I think, like I said, not just Tourette's but with any disability. I think we're showing them, because were older, so we're able to verbalize what the children may be going through. (Tracey 333-340)

Mike also believes there are strengths when working with families as well:

A lot of times families want me to be an advocate for their kid. I struggle with that for two reasons. First of all, I can't get to the meetings because I'm at school the same time they are having their meeting, and I just can't take off and do that. But I can just give them reassurance that, "Yeah, it's your kid and do what's best for them," and I think that that's the most important thing. And I think that some people think that if the teacher says that, they have to do it, and that's not necessarily the case. Sometimes teachers just don't understand yet, and it takes a little bit of time. I always tell the parents to allow them that time, but also give them the resources and strategies to help them and help the child be successful. (Mike 283 – 290)

Sue believes there are strengths when working with families as well:

I think some of the same kind of things. I think I understand, and probably not just from teaching but from running the chapter, the state chapter, for so many years that parents have to go through a grieving process. And I saw this with a kid that I was teaching. If a child would be diagnosed with something, whether it be a learning disability, a neurological disorder, a physical illness, a lot of times parents just have to have time to absorb all that and become used to that. And I think especially with Tourette because it's one of those lifelong disorders. When you tell a parent of a six-year-old, "Your kid's got Tourette and that's it." It's also a very unpredictable disorder. We don't know what route it's going to take, at any moment, at any given time. I think you can sort of understand it from a parent's point of view, how difficult that is to accept that kind of thing for a child. I think, because of not only teaching but also working with, and I think parents, especially of kids with special needs, I could talk to them in a more personal way than a teacher who had never had a disability herself, nor had a child with one. Because they didn't know what that experience was like. And not only do I have it myself, but I have many, many family members with it. Every time a relative, a child is diagnosed in our family, we all kind of go through a grieving process, even though we all know what it is, we understand it, we know that help is out there, but it's still difficult. I think I'm more able to relate a little bit to the parents. I had a call the other day from a parent who has been absolutely, her child is a sixth grader, and she just doesn't want to classify him. The school had me come in and observe him, and it was so obvious that as bright as he was, he did need some services, things like testing in a separate location, just little things. The parent had been absolutely refusing it, and I got onto the phone, and I talked to her for about a half-hour, 45 minutes, and by the time I finished, she was like, "When can we sign up for this?" And I think she took it better from me because I was a teacher, so I understand education, but I have Tourette. I have a disability. I have this myself, and she was much more capable, maybe I was able to explain it to her better than if it was coming from the teachers, who

were maybe a little more judgmental. I don't know.
I don't know exactly what it is, but I think it does
make it easier to work with families in a lot of
ways. And I think also, you probably know just
from personal experience, parents are always
judged by their kids' behavior. And if you've got a
child who's got these disorders and nobody knows
that they have these disorders, then you're always
looked at as the parent who can't make their kids
behave. "Why is your child always doing this?"
"Why are they always making these noises?" Or
whatever. As a person with this disorder, I kind of
look at the parents differently. I know it's not your
fault that this has happened to your child. You spent
a lifetime, you've spent years now blaming yourself,
and it's not really your fault. And I think that that
helps a lot. Because parents get sick of being
blamed. I know it's not your fault. Like I'm sure this
teacher today was thinking, "This kid is attention
seeking, he must not get a lot of attention at home.
Otherwise he wouldn't be so attention seeking."
That's our immediate judgment call. And I can look
at him and think, "Hmm, I don't think this has
anything to do with seeking attention. This is just
neurological. Why would he want to seek attention
in this way? It's so embarrassing for him. It's
terrible." (Sue 718 – 756)

Sue believed having Tourette syndrome is an asset when
working with families.

I think it's a great asset. But I think if anything else
in my life, it was an asset for me to be able to work
with parents. They found me to be more
compassionate and understanding of their kids,
willing to try different things and willing to go that
extra step or extra mile for them because I
understood them. There were things that were

harder for these kids. Life was just going to be harder. And I also think that a lot of families probably saw me as a role model for their kids who have disabilities. And I think that's a real important thing too. That they can see that it is bad, I have actually had kids that say that to me. Like, "I see how well that you did, so I'm not going to let my disability get me down." And it makes me feel fantastic. There's nothing more rewarding coming from a kid than to have somebody say that. Many times kids would say that to me when they would get down about their disability or whatever it was they were dealing with. But I think with families, they kind of have this sense that you understood. That you understood their child. And even though every kid who you teach is different, and they knew that you had this understanding that these aren't just all little robots sitting in front of you here, and everybody learning exactly the same way. We do it this way and this way, and we do things that way. Teachers can become very rigid, as you probably know. I think I never was that kind of person. And I know it sounds like I'm attributing a lot to this, but I think really when you deal with something like this your whole life, those are the things you learn. And not only about yourself and about other kids. And in some ways, it was a help for me. (Sue 831 – 861)

Challenges Due to Disclosing

However, Laura knows there can also be challenges when working with students and identifying as an educator with Tourette syndrome:

Well, that first couple weeks before I tell them, they're always kind of looking at you like, "What are you doing?" And, "Why are you doing that?" And they don't, as much as they want to, they don't always understand. So they may not understand you're having a bad day with your tics. And they don't really understand why. You can't talk to your students about everything. (Laura 309 – 312)

There are also challenges when working with families:

Parent teacher conferences are a little bit embarrassing sometimes. Especially with the parents I don't know as well, I'm always afraid I'm going to start ticcing out of control, and they are going to be like, "What is wrong with my child's teacher?" But usually, it turned out okay. (Laura 320 – 322)

Tracey knows there can be challenges in being an educator with Tourette syndrome:

The challenges, I think, well sometimes I think just the tics themselves can be challenging in general. I think we're all human, and sometimes you do have the tendency to be a little impatient with your students. And sometimes you don't understand. Just because we have Tourette's doesn't mean we understand what all children are going through. You don't understand what they may be dealing with in regards to ADHD or things of that nature. I think that sometimes the challenge is that: patience and caring and trying to put yourself where the children are coming from. (Tracey 348 – 354)

Challenges arise when working with parents as well:

You know what, working with parents themselves, I'm sure you know this, can be difficult in general.

Parents don't always know where you're coming from. And I think as a person, I sometimes can get very impatient with parents when they don't understand what I'm trying to say to them. And I think that, especially with having the OCD, you want things a certain way, you feel like you have to do things. And parents don't always understand that. They expect you sometimes to be on their schedule. So I really think that's hard explaining to parents why you are the way you are. Why you have to do things, and doing your job, plus having all those quirks. (Tracey 357 – 363)

Sue acknowledges that there can also be challenges in identifying as an educator with Tourette syndrome:

I suppose just them not understanding. It's going to be an issue at some point. I think, in my opinion, it's up to you how much of an issue you want to make it. Those first few days of school, of course, once I knew what I had, it made a big difference, but kids are kids. They're going to invariably ask, "Why do you do that?" I go in and observe classes now and people ask me. Kids will ask me. They'll imitate my tics. They are not doing it to be mean, it's just peculiar to them. Why does she keep doing that? So at some point, especially at the beginning of the school year, it is going to be an issue, and then I think it's all in how much of an issue you make it. I never used it as an excuse. It was a reason why sometimes I had to do certain things, but it was never an excuse for not doing my job, for not caring about kids, or not teaching my subject matter. And I would immediately deal with it at the beginning of the year by, I would tell them what it was, give them a kind of brief overview in language they could understand, so they knew what it was. And then I would say, "I don't think it's going to be an issue, now you understand it," and that's kind of the end of it. Life goes on, and I think I just never wanted it to be who I was. And I didn't want them to go home and say, "I have this teacher with Tourette." I wanted them to go home and say, "I have this teacher who's a good teacher. I have a teacher who does fun things with us." I didn't want that to identify who I was. So I just made it as little of an issue as I could. And sometimes there are things you have to deal with, but I think some people just, I'm not saying they make more out of it than they have to but that I think sometimes it doesn't have to be the biggest issue if you just deal with it upfront. I found sometimes joking with the kids about it. And I would say to them after I would joke about it, "It's not really fun to live with. It's not something that's funny, but this is how I've survived it." It eases their comfort level. Because I think there's a little bit on the part of kids and other staff members of embarrassment for you. And once they know that I'm not embarrassed by it anymore, even though there are many times that I am, it's okay. I'm okay with this. And I think that they're more at ease with it. And they know that it's something you can joke about, and that's the end of it. I'm not going to make a big deal out of it. If somebody would bring it up again I'd say, "Remember I have that thing called Tourette syndrome. I talked to you about that earlier, and that's why I do these things." And that's the end of it. I just never wanted it to be a huge issue in my classroom. I just didn't want that to happen. I didn't want to be a teacher who has Tourette or tics. I'm just a teacher. And I come here to teach kids. I don't worry about having Tourette. (Sue 800 – 829)

Stacy feels that sometimes having Tourette can get in the way of her teaching:

Sometimes I find I don't get my point across, I'm not very clear. I get distracted I guess. I get focused on suppressing the tics. (Stacy 108 – 109)

She views this as a challenge of being a teacher with Tourette syndrome:

Sometimes I am so self-aware of how the students are perceiving me in the classroom and if they see me tic, that I lose focus on the real purpose that I am there which is to be their teacher. Like if I'm trying to explain a point and I'm ticcing, I become aware of that and lose my train of thought. (Stacy 162 – 165)

Empowerment in Disclosing

It seems that the positives outweighed the negatives for Laura. She felt a sense of empowerment in disclosing at work:

It kind of let me say, "My Tourette's doesn't rule me. It's not something to be ashamed of. It's not something that defines who I am." By identifying it, it's just like saying, "Hey, whatever, I've got this. It's not me. I'm not Tourette's. I am a teacher who has Tourette's." (Laura 328 – 330)

Disclosing at work has empowered Michelle:

I didn't realize that I was uncomfortable before. And I think I've discovered that now that I am letting myself tic during the day, I think I'm definitely more comfortable, and I don't have to think about where I'm going to sit in the room necessarily and those types of things. I know that if it's a really stressful day, and I know I'm going to tic more, it's okay if I tic in front of people. (Michelle 364 – 367)

Tracey does believe disclosing at work has empowered her:

> I feel a little bit more free to be myself. I don't feel
> as bottled up. When you don't tell people you have
> Tourette's, you're afraid to tic, you're afraid to let
> yourself shine through. You spend all day
> suppressing those tics and making excuses for why
> you do things. You know, when I didn't disclose my
> first year, children would, "Mrs. Miller, why are
> you making that noise?" "Oh no, no, no, it's just a
> habit." And I think you spend so much time making
> excuses for your behavior, whereas when you tell
> people what you have, it's just much easier to say,
> as you know, "That's just a tic." And I also feel like
> it's more educating for them because we're not
> hiding from them what's going on. We're showing
> them and telling them that this is a real disorder out
> there, and explaining to them, and they are learning.
> So I definitely think it helps me to be more myself.
> (Tracey 374 – 383)

She does not feel like disclosing has constrained her at all:

> I don't feel like it has constrained me by any means.
> I really feel, I don't feel that people look at me
> differently. I do feel people are more understanding
> and definitely can adapt better. So I really feel like
> it's probably the best thing that I've ever done.
> (Tracey 385 – 387)

Mike also believes disclosing at school has empowered him:

> If I didn't, I wouldn't be me. Tourette's syndrome is
> part of who I am. So if the school can't accept it,
> then I'm not going to be able to be an effective
> teacher. That's pretty simple for me. I disclose so I
> am able to be who I am. That makes me able to
> share my strengths with the community, and that's a
> good thing. (Mike 292 – 295)

Disclosing at work empowered Sue:

> Oh, it's huge. It's no longer the big secret. There's a
> new commercial out for, I think it might be for
> insurance or something, where the guy's walking
> around, I always love this. He's got two huge
> weights around his neck, and all the sudden he just
> drops them. That's what it felt like to let everybody
> know I had Tourette. It's like the weight of the
> world is off your shoulders. Because you're always
> looking around, "Who's noticing?" Every day, there
> was not a day that went by that I wasn't worried
> about who was thinking, what they were thinking,
> did they think I was just crazy, did they think I was
> very nervous, what were the kids thinking? And
> you tried your best, but it was horrible. So I think
> just knowing what it was and disclosing and letting
> people know was like, "Wow. This is great, I can
> just be me, and I don't have to worry about it
> anymore." It was huge. And I think many, many,
> many kids feel the same way. Although I'd
> encounter a lot of parents who don't want other
> people to know. More because of themselves than
> their child. But the kids are so relieved when
> everybody knows. Now they know why I'm doing
> it, they don't just think I'm the weird kid in class. I
> don't have to sit here and try to suppress for 45
> minutes. It really is a huge weight off your
> shoulders. Definitely. (Sue 917 – 930)

She does not think it constrained her at all:

> I don't think it did it all. I can't think of any ways. I
> think it was, everybody knows, and each year you'd
> encounter new staff members that would come in,
> and I think I told you about the one that asked me if
> I taught sign language because I have a lot of finger
> tics. And you have to explain all over again, but

once it's done, it's done. That's the end of it. And people just don't even pay attention to it anymore. I didn't find any constraints at all. And it was the best thing that ever happened to me. That I was finally diagnosed. (Sue 932 – 937)

Disclosing at work has been empowering for me as well. The more open I am about Tourette, the more accepting my students are.

Understanding for Students with Special Needs

Laura feels like she has a greater understanding for students with special needs or students going through a difficult time because of having Tourette:

Absolutely. I would have teachers that wouldn't understand, "I don't want to sit in the front of the class." And they'd be like, "Tough, suck it up." Just things like that. I can understand when kids just need something different. I know that it's not really just them being difficult, they really do need it. And so I feel like I'm more sympathetic towards them and can put myself in their shoes more. (Laura 344 – 347)

Michelle also feels like she understands students with special needs better because of having Tourette syndrome:

I think I probably do. I don't think about it that way, on a daily basis. But I think that I definitely do. As far as, especially the kids at the language end piece of it, the kids that are probably going to be identified as learning disabled along the road. Again, this whole executive functioning piece because that's something that really affects me. Teaching kids how to cope with that, how to get around it sort of. "Adults make lists, it's okay for kids to make lists." That type of thing. Helping to give ideas for organizing themselves in the classroom, whatnot. I think that that's helped a lot. (Michelle 378 – 384)

Jason also feels like he understands students with special needs better because he is an educator with Tourette syndrome:

Absolutely, absolutely. Like I said working at a former school, when I worked there, I didn't even know. I knew I had something different about me. It helped me to understand after I found out what I had, why those kids that are a little bit different and the troubles that they are going through and the problems they are going through, not being able to do what I expected of them, it helped me understand that they've got other things going on. Other than, "Hey, I need you to learn this." They've got some other stuff to overcome. (Jason 353 – 358)

Tracey also feels like she understands students with special needs or students going through a difficult time because of having Tourette syndrome:

I do. I wouldn't say that I understand all disabilities or that having a child with a disability is not challenging. My sister has three children who are all autistic. And I feel like I can be more understanding to her and understanding to the kids, but I don't feel like I understand all the disabilities. But I do feel that having a disability makes me a little bit more compassionate and understanding and patient. And also it's sympathetic. And when a child has a disability, coming from someone that does, I want to know all and learn all I can about that disability. Because I don't want to make assumptions about them. I don't want to downgrade them or put my standards too high for them. So I really feel that a lot of people, until you have a child with a disability or you have a disability, I do feel like sometimes we aren't as compassionate to those students. So I do feel like it's helped out a lot. (Tracey 399 – 408)

Mike, too, believes he understands students with special needs better because of having Tourette:

Absolutely. I've been there. And I can relate to some of their struggles that they may have. Not only that but it's not just that I can relate to their struggles, but I like to think that I can help them get over that hump. Sometimes it just takes that little extra push. Hopefully I'll be able to give that to them. (Mike 309 – 312)

Sue definitely feels she understands students with special needs better because of having Tourette syndrome:

Absolutely. Absolutely. 100 percent. There's no question in my mind. I only wish I had known about, I mean I knew I had something, but I wish early on I'd known what I had because I can think of kids that I taught years ago who probably had Tourette, but I never knew what it was because I didn't know what I had. But boy, certainly. Kids don't come to school every day and say, "I'm coming here to fail today." It's not their purpose in life. Kids will do well if they can. And that's the honest to God truth, and I think somebody has to be in their corner. 100 percent, it changed my whole style of teaching, my empathy towards kids, I mean everything I think was, having Tourette made me so much stronger as a teacher, so much better a teacher. Definitely. I think most teachers who have

Tourette would probably tell you that. (Sue 959 – 967)

Stacy feels like she is able to question what is going on with a student if problems occur in the classroom. She feels like this helps her reach students with special needs because she does not let them slip through the cracks.

I agree with my participants that I have a better understanding of students with special needs because I have Tourette. I am empathetic with other students because I have been there before. I understand what they're going through.

Conclusion

Even though not all of my participants openly disclosed to students, many have had positive experiences when they did disclose. Many participants have found that there are strengths in identifying as an educator with Tourette syndrome. It is not always an easy road, but it has proved for many to be beneficial. Just as there are strengths, there are also challenges with identifying as an educator with Tourette syndrome. Despite the challenges, participants felt a feeling of empowerment in disclosing to their students. In doing this, they answered questions about Tourette as openly and honestly as possible. All participants felt they understood students with special needs better because they have a disability themselves. Many participants stated that having Tourette syndrome made them more compassionate, understanding, and sympathetic teachers.

CHAPTER SEVEN

WHAT IT MEANS TO BE AN EDUCATOR WITH TOURETTE SYNDROME

Purpose

In this chapter, I will examine the meaning that participants make out of being an educator with Tourette syndrome. I focused on four main questions: 1) What is it like to be an educator with Tourette syndrome? 2) What does it mean to be an educator with Tourette syndrome? 3) What are some of the hidden rules or expectations you are expected to follow as an educator with Tourette syndrome? 4) How does having Tourette syndrome shape your life? Five common themes were apparent in the meaning participants made out of being an educator with Tourette syndrome. They were: 1) being an educator with Tourette syndrome is difficult, 2) being an educator with Tourette syndrome does not mean anything different from being an educator, 3) they are called upon to educate others and assist others in similar situations, 4) there are hidden rules and expectations we are expected to follow, and 5) there is information others need to know about being an educator with Tourette syndrome. I will explore these themes in detail in this chapter.

Being an Educator with Tourette Syndrome Is Difficult

The participants in my study reflect on what it is like to be an educator with Tourette syndrome. Laura notes that being an educator with Tourette syndrome can be difficult:

It's a little bit frustrating. It's just one extra thing we have to deal with, especially since this was my first year. It's kind of annoying that I had to take time out of class to talk about it. That I had to explain to new colleagues what was happening. But on the other hand, it's kind of neat because it teaches kids acceptance. It really was a bonding experience for my class. (Laura 206 – 209)

Tracey talks about what it is like to be an educator with Tourette syndrome. She, like Laura, notes the different difficulties:

It's very difficult because especially with the kids you know, even though you explain it to them, you know that they're looking at you and that they're watching your moves. And it is hard sometimes when I'm trying to make a point and I'm shaking my head, and I think sometimes they do get confused like, "Oh, was that a tic, or is she doing something different?" And you feel like when you're in staff meetings, sometimes I do feel like people are watching me, even though I'm sure that they're not. You tend to feel that they are. And when you have report card night and conferences with parents, I feel very uncomfortable and self-conscious ticcing in front of them, and I try not to but sometimes you can't always hold it in. It's just very, like I said, I think that I'm always self-conscious that people are watching me and judging me. It's very hard and difficult with the OCD, just getting to school in the morning or getting distracted, having that routine, sometimes I feel like I need extra time for things because I'm spending my day focusing, dealing with myself. (Tracey 191 – 202)

Being an Educator with Tourette Syndrome Does Not Mean Anything Different from Being an Educator

Michelle reflects on what it is like to be an educator with Tourette syndrome. For her, it is a positive experience:

> I think in the beginning, it was hard for me because I was actively trying to hide it. But I think now, I don't think it's hard. I think it's kind of cool actually. Because when the kids have heard about it or learn about it, it gives me an opportunity to explain it. So I kind of like that that's changed over the last year. There definitely is, the older the kids are, the more intimidated I am by it. Just because, kids are cruel. So you don't really know, particularly with fifth-graders, what's going to happen. But I think it's kind of cool to have the opportunity to teach them and hope that they go home and talk to their parents about it is really what I would love to see happen. (Michelle 231 – 237)

Michelle comments on what it means to be an educator with Tourette syndrome. She believes it is great that people with disabilities are becoming successful educators:

> I think it means that anybody can really go into the field. It doesn't affect me as much, but for other people that are really affected by it, it's a big thing. It's something that people notice right away. And I think it's great for kids and parents to see that anybody can be a teacher. (Michelle 327 – 329)

Jason also talks about what it is like to be an educator with Tourette syndrome:

> I guess just the same as a teacher without. I think I have a view of kids with different disabilities, learning disabilities. I have a better view, I think, than a teacher who doesn't have any disabilities

because I have to overcome the whole tic thing and the obsessive compulsiveness because as a teacher, you can't have your room completely neat and orderly all the time, and I have to overcome that. And there are certain boundaries that I have to overcome that other teachers don't have to. And I can understand why some kids don't learn at the same rate as others because they have other things going on. (Jason 277 – 283)

Mike discusses what it is like to be an educator with Tourette syndrome. Like Michelle, he focuses on the positives:

I love it. I was different, you know. I was special. I never had the problem with the weight on my shoulder to be the role model. I always felt like I was a role model for kids that had special needs or maybe that are just average. I think so many times we have role models out there that are sports athletes and or actors and actresses. They are people that are so distant. I think that sometimes a role model should be people who are closest to our lives, like our parents or family members, or our teachers and educators. I had no problem with it. I just tried to show kids that this is what I have. You may not have chosen the disability or weakness that you have in life. I definitely didn't choose mine. But you just have to accept it, and if you choose not to accept it, you're going to go down a different road. And that's a road that I just didn't want to go down. So I just tried to be the role model for some of the young people out there. (Mike 217 – 226)

Stacy reflects on what it is like to be an educator with Tourette syndrome:

I don't know if it's much different. As an educator, I wonder if some of the kids notice. I'm sure they do.

> But most people say I'm a pretty quirky person. But I've definitely had little kids, like kindergartners, ask, "Why do you do that?" Which is slightly awkward. And I'm not very good at explaining it. I'll say, "Oh, I was itching my eye." I don't know if it creates a whole lot of difficulty. It's hard having people around you all the time when you want to get it out of your system. So sometimes I like having my breaks, where I need to be alone in my room. Because having a lot of people, sometimes I have sixty kids in my room and having that many eyes on you is hard. Otherwise, I don't have a whole lot of issues. (Stacy 99 – 106)

Similarly, Laura talks about what it means to be an educator with Tourette syndrome:

> I don't think it really means anything different than just being an educator. My Tourette's isn't who I am. It's something I deal with, something I'll always deal with, but it doesn't have to define me, and it doesn't define my career. (Laura 284 – 286)

Sue reflects on what it means to be an educator with Tourette syndrome. Her response is similar to Laura's:

> I don't think it's any different than being an educator. I'm a teacher; I teach kids certain subject areas. The fact that I have Tourette, to me, is unimportant. I don't think it's an issue. It never has been. (Sue 668 – 670)

We Are Called Upon to Educate Others and Assist in Similar Situations

Sue reflects on what it is like to be an educator with Tourette syndrome. She recalls how having Tourette syndrome made her a better teacher:

> Well it's, I don't think it has to be any different than any another educator. I've always said to people I have Tourette; it's not who I am. And that's just something I've always kind of maintained. I say this in all honesty, it really made me a better teacher. Because I could see kids, and I could see that sometimes there are just things that, like when you've got your little hyperactive child who just can't sit still, rather than every two seconds yelling at him, let's figure out a way. This kid can't sit still, so let's figure out a way. Let's find a place in the room for him or send him on a little errand, let them pass out papers, erase the board, whatever it is that you have to do. Because you look at this kid instead of just being mad at him or yelling at him and embarrassing him for something he has no control over. I think it really made me a much, much better teacher. But yet it wasn't, it wasn't really, I don't ever see that it interfered with my teaching. I don't think. I never did. I think I was probably not the same teacher I would have been if I didn't have it. I have it. I think I was probably a better teacher with having it. But it really didn't change my teaching at all. I've always said anybody can do whatever they want to do. It doesn't make any difference if they have Tourette. I had a mother who asked me, going back about eight or nine years now, and her son, they were Catholic, and her son was an altar boy, or wanted to be an altar boy but he had coprolalia, and she was really worried about that. And she said, "I've had to tell him no. You just can't do it. There's

some things you won't be able to do." And I said to her, "You spent your life telling him that he can do whatever he wants to do, that Tourette doesn't have to stop him. And now you're telling him he can't be an altar boy because he has Tourette. So you're kind of going against what you told him all along." She said, "Well, how can I let him get up on the altar and be yelling, 'Fuck you,' to the congregation?" And I said, "Well, what do we do in any situation? We educate people." So I went in with her we got up in front of the Mass he was going to serve. And it was usually the same people mostly every week, and we did a little 10 minute deal on Tourette. The priest let us do it, and he continued to serve mass and yell the F- word. It was just not a big deal. And I think that's kind of the attitude you have to have. (Sue 405 – 430)

Tracey talks about what it means to be an educator with Tourette syndrome. She thinks it is crucial to use her role as an educator to educate others on the disability:

I think it has a lot to do with educating other people. I think the benefit of being a teacher is that we can educate kids and parents and other employees about Tourette's. I think as a teacher, it helps you because you know the right way to teach them. (Tracey 324 – 326)

Hidden Rules and Expectations We Are Expected to Follow

Laura discusses some of the hidden rules and expectations she is expected to follow as an educator with Tourette syndrome:

Well I mean, obviously, it would be not really acceptable if I started shouting random words in

class or during meetings or at a parent teacher
conference or something. But I think mostly that
my administration had never dealt with it before, so
we were kind of just following it together to see
what happened. And it really worked out okay.
(Laura 272 – 275)

Michelle discusses some of the hidden rules or expectations
she is expected to follow as an educator with Tourette
syndrome. She focuses on the rules she's made for herself:

I don't think they have rules; I think I've set my own
rules. Well again, how I would hide it all the time.
When my kids were diagnosed, I would talk about it
in terms of my kids, but I really didn't talk about in
terms of myself, until just this past year or so. So I
think that's a rule I made for myself. Positioning
myself in the room. Again as far as where my desk
was before and where my desk is now. Just
knowing where people were. And even still, if I go
to the lunch room or faculty meetings, I always
position myself in the back. I don't know if that's
consciously a Tourette's related decision, but my
whole life I've done that. Even in college, when I
was taking classes, I was always in the back of the
room. So again I don't know if that was a conscious
Tourette's decision, but I am always a back of the
room person. Or facing the door person. (Michelle
304 – 312)

Jason mentions the hidden rules or expectations he is
expected to follow as an educator with Tourette syndrome. He
discusses being a liaison for his administrators:

I think the education value. I think if it comes up
again with a student at another school, I think
there's probably an expectation that the
superintendent might say, "Jason Marks, let's

contact him and see if he can help us out with it."
I've had the mother of that student, he actually left
and went to another school a year or so later, and
she's called on me a couple of times to help out his
new teachers. So I think it's just the education
value. (Jason 332 – 336)

Tracey discusses some of the hidden rules or expectations
she is expected to follow as an educator with Tourette
syndrome. She mentions the extra steps an educator with
Tourette syndrome has to take in order to be a successful
teacher:

I don't know that there are necessarily any hidden
rules that we're expected to follow. I think that
sometimes people don't understand how difficult it
is for us. It's not as simple as just coming into
school in the morning and teaching. Our tics
sometimes, you're ticcing so bad, you can't focus on
the task at hand. I find that if I'm really, really
nervous, I tic uncontrollably. And that makes it hard
to teach and that makes it hard to get your work
done. And a lot of children and adults with
Tourette's syndrome have the ADHD with that or
they have the OCD and with that is a whole other
set of problems. I don't think that more is expected
of us, other than to be understanding, but I do feel
like people don't understand how much harder it is
for us as an educator. (Tracey 288 – 295)

Sue talks about some of the hidden rules or expectations she
is expected to follow as an educator with Tourette syndrome:

I think the one really problem area was the
coprolalia. Because that's something they don't
expect you to do. They don't want you to do that in
a school setting. I had to figure out a way, and I
think I pretty successfully did that. I turned to the

blackboard. I remember one time years ago though, there was a show called *The Geraldo Show*. Geraldo Rivera, and I was a guest on his program. He did one of the best shows ever on Tourette many years ago, which was surprising knowing Geraldo. He asked me that very question. And I said when I have to swear, I turned to the blackboard and try to say it under my breath or muffle it so nobody understands it. And then I remember saying to him, "The fact that I just told this on national television probably isn't going to help, is it?" When I got back to my classroom, every time I turned to the board, one of my kids would say, "Are you swearing?" I used to always say, "You'll never know." And so it got to be kind of a joke with the kids. I think you just knew there were certain things, especially before I was diagnosed, that you didn't want. I knew once I was diagnosed that they didn't really have a right to fire me for the coprolalia. But it's not something I personally wanted the kids to hear. So I really worked at it. And to this day I can muffle it so that nobody really hears what I'm saying, and I find ways of camouflaging it. I can't think of anything else really. I think one of the biggest challenges was each year, as new teachers came in that didn't know you. I was in the staff room one morning a couple years before I retired, and one of the newly hired special education teachers came up to me, and she looked at me and she said, "Hi, my name is Melissa, I bet you teach sign language." Because I have a lot of hand tics, my hands are always moving, and of course everybody else in the room was like, [inhales breath]. And I looked at her and I said, "No, but I'd sure confuse those little deaf children, wouldn't I?" And everybody was relieved and realized that I could just make a joke out of it. Then I said to her, "I have Tourette syndrome." She was just so embarrassed and apologized to me every day for weeks. Finally I just said, "Melissa, really, if that's the only thing that anybody's ever said to me in my life, that would be good. Really, don't worry about it. Stop apologizing. I'm fine with it." Because it does look weird, and that's what you would think. Those kinds of things, new teachers and being observed was always a little difficult. They have to come observe you, and I could be a challenge. But otherwise, I was just myself, good, bad, or otherwise. (Sue 594 – 621)

What Others Need to Know About Being an Educator with Tourette Syndrome

Laura discusses how Tourette syndrome does not need to be a taboo subject at work. What Laura most wants people to know about being an educator with Tourette syndrome is:

I guess just that once I start ticcing in front of colleagues, it just gets worse and worse because I get embarrassed about the initial tics. And so then they keep happening. I basically just want people to know it's okay to say, "I see that your Tourette's is really bad right now. Are you okay?" It's okay to talk about it and not just ignore it and act like it's something that we can't ever mention. It's okay to acknowledge it. (Laura 278 – 282)

Laura also discusses the lack of knowledge about Tourette syndrome:

I guess I just wish there was more education out there about it. It has such a stigma still, you know the coprolalia and people yelling cuss words. And I'm like, no, that's not, I mean some people do that, but I don't do that. I guess I wish it was more like

ADHD or something that people just knew what it was and were like, okay, and accepted it. (Laura 367 – 370)

Tracey wants others to know this about people with Tourette syndrome:

> I think the point I wanted to get across is we're just like everybody else, but sometimes it's a little bit more difficult, which I really think that you're going to portray very well in your book. It's funny because we are not, I don't think, handicapped. I think it's nice to see that we're becoming teachers. I think that it's wonderful that you're bringing awareness to this cause. And another teacher with Tourette's that has written a book, how he went on to be a wonderful teacher and a great speaker. And it's nice to see that, although it's not always easy for us, it's difficult, we really can strive and really do well for ourselves. And I think that's important because it's hard to be a teacher in general, but when you have any kind of disability, I think it makes it even more difficult. So to see a lot of people out there with all these disabilities, to see them striving and becoming teachers and really good teachers, I think that's really impressive. (Tracey 443 – 452)

Mike discusses how it's okay to be a person with a disability. He also mentions people have to respect other's privacy and the ways people with disabilities choose to disclose or not disclose. Mike wants others to know this about people with Tourette syndrome:

> Everybody with Tourette's is a little different. For me, I have loud vocal tics and so I couldn't hide that. For me, I couldn't suppress. I mean, how do you camouflage a loud barking sound? But I don't

ever judge people who say, "I didn't want to disclose," or, "I didn't want to share." Because even though we all have Tourette's, even though we're all part of that special club, we're still different. We're still ourselves. One has to figure out how we're going to deal with life in our own way. One person with a loud vocal tic and another person who just has crazy eye twitches or some other stuff, it's a lot different in how you want to handle it. So you have to respect that too. (Mike 336 – 342)

Sue is truly an inspiring woman. She wants people to know this about Tourette syndrome:

It's always been a challenge, and I'll admit it. It's just one more thing you have to think about and worry about. But you can't, I learned early on, that you can't let it take over your life and ruin your career or take over your dreams and what you really want to do in life. And I see so many people with Tourette who have been so successful because they've had a positive attitude about it. And I think that's kind of always what I wanted to do. To me, it's all in how you look at it, adjust to it, deal with it in society. I go to support group meetings; I run a support group meeting here. As a matter of fact, it was so interesting because I got a phone call three weeks ago from a girl who is actually one of my students who I taught probably 15 years ago, maybe more than that now. She left my class in eighth grade; I had her for three years. She went on to high school, and as a junior in high school, she was diagnosed with Tourette. She didn't actually start with her symptoms until she was 15, which is very unusual, as you know. Hardly anybody starts that late in life. She ended up coming to our last support group meeting that I was running. It's so interesting because she started so late in life and had some pretty negative experiences with jobs and college. And her attitude is really kind of down right now. Her whole demeanor is. She's not working, she's married, and her husband works, so she has support. She's trying to collect disability. I think part of her problem is just the way she's looking at this whole thing. Maybe because she started so late in life and didn't really have time to adjust. I can't think of a worse age than 15 to start with Tourette. That is such a critical age for kids. After meeting with us, I hooked her up with a counselor. She's called me a few times, we've had some great chats, we went out for coffee, and I'm starting to see everything change. I'm starting to see her look at life a little bit differently. I think it's helping her in the long run. You see that, and I can understand how people get there. I definitely can. But I think when she came to her meeting, she walked into her meeting, and she sat down, and she said, "One of the best things that happened at this meeting is we all laughed. Some parents cried, and then they laughed. Then they cried, then they laughed." She said, "I was crying, and I was laughing." And she said, "I think you have to see that you can do both when you have Tourette or when you have a child with Tourette." There will be times when you are going to cry. The pain gets to you and everything else, but let's face it, it can be hysterical. Some of the bizarre situations you get yourself into, you just have to be like, "Oh my God, this is so ridiculous." I think attitude is everything. And I think if you look at a situation like Tourette isn't that big of a deal to you, then that's how your students look at it. And after a while, they just don't notice it. They know you for you and not for the tics. You can imagine, when you think back to teachers that you had, growing up, that you hated because of their mean, negative attitude who would embarrass the kids. If they had Tourette, oh my God. That would be something that kids would be relentless with. And so I think I knew, at the very beginning, especially with middle school kids who can be a lot that way anyway, if I didn't get them on my side that first couple days of school every year, it was done for the year. So those first few days were absolutely critical to me. And to try to get them to see me for me and not for the tics. To let them know who I was, and that I did have a sense of humor, and I was going to understand them, and they were going to be safe in my room. And I think that made a huge difference. But I could see if I had a teacher like some of the teachers that I've met going into schools, and if they had Tourette; oh boy, we could've had a field day. (Sue 624 – 665)

Sue also wants people to understand:

It's an interesting journey. And I think anybody who has Tourette, like yourself, can tell you there's not a day that somebody doesn't say something to you about it. Everywhere you go, people have said to me sometimes, "Don't you get tired of the staring?" Because I'm sure, when you're out, people stare. And they do. And I'll kind of look out of the corner of my eye, and I've got three kids kind of glaring at me. And you want to go, "Excuse me, is there a problem?" But I think that part of it, you just kind of get used to. You just get used to learning to tell people what it is, now that I know. But it is hurtful at times. There are many, many times I've been very hurt by it. And many times that I've been asked to leave places, and I knew it wasn't fair, but what are you going to do? This is just the way life is. I think one of the things I used to tell my students all the time, life is not fair. What's fair is not always equal, and what is equal is not always fair. That's just the way life is. We do our best, but it's not perfect. So I guess it's just one of those things, it's something that I have spent a life trying to get used to, but despite that fact, there are still days when it gets old. When it just gets old. And it's like, could I just have ten minutes, that's all I want. Ten minutes without ticcing. It's always going to be a challenge. I had a principal one time who said to me, if I can get this quote right, "Life is ten percent what happens to you and ninety percent what you do about it." And I absolutely love that quote. I don't know where she got it from, but it's true. This is what happened to me. I got Tourette and a few dozen other things, but now what do I do with it? Do I let it ruin me? And stay home and not see the world and do whatever I want to do? Or do I just go out there and say listen, this is me and this is who I am, and if you don't like it, well I guess you don't have to hang around with me. And just go for your dreams and do what you want to do in life. (Sue 1058 – 1078)

Conclusion

Participants described how being an educator with a disability is more difficult than just being an educator. Some of the participants were self-conscious of their tics and worried that others were watching them and judging them. At the same time, it teaches kids acceptance. Being an educator with Tourette gives us the opportunity to explain it and educate others. Many of the participants felt that they are more understanding than teachers who do not have any disabilities.

Some participants felt like they are a role model for kids who have special needs or even kids who are just average. One teacher said her Tourette isn't who she is. It is a part of her, yes, but it doesn't define her or her career. Other teachers discussed how although it is not always easy for educators with Tourette, we can accomplish great things in our lives. Even though Tourette can be a challenge, we're not going to let it take over our lives or ruin our career. Despite having Tourette, these educators successfully and competently balanced the pressures and demands of being an educator along with having Tourette syndrome.

CHAPTER EIGHT

THRIVING WITH TOURETTE SYNDROME

Discussion of Results

Participants in this research embraced their disability. In doing so, certain themes became apparent about the lives of these seven educators. Disclosing to administrators, colleagues, students and their parents, and personal friends was a positive experience. Participants found numerous strengths in disclosing to others. One such strength was the fact that people were extremely accepting of them once they were educated about Tourette syndrome. Embracing their disability was empowering not only to my participants, but also to me. Being a teacher with Tourette syndrome is not any different from being a teacher. These people are not only surviving at being educators, they are thriving at it. One asset they have is that their disability has made them more compassionate and understanding to students with special needs or students going through a difficult time.

Through the portrayal of these seven educators, I have provided my readers with a glimpse of what life is like for an educator with Tourette syndrome. In looking at life through the lens of educators with Tourette syndrome, one is able to see that being an educator with a disability is not easy. "If I was going to exist with any degree of dignity and independence, then I had no choice but to prove that Tourette syndrome would never get the best of me" (Cohen, 2005, p. 128). Despite obstacles, these educators have persevered and become successful teachers. "We all play the hand we are dealt, and we all choose how we'll live" (Cohen, 2005, p. 221). It is my hope that the lived experiences of these educators with a disability, in this case Tourette syndrome, will encourage administrators to actively recruit educators with disabilities for their school districts. Administrators need to do so, as there are few educators with disabilities in the profession. The significantly low representation of people with disabilities in academic settings, in positions as students, faculty, and administrators, has excluded their voice in discussions on curricular reform (Longmore & Umansky, 2001).

Summary of the Study

This research was the combination of a phenomenological study and an autoethnography. As there is no research on educators with Tourette syndrome, I wanted to build the foundation of that knowledge base. I used phenomenological research techniques to interview seven other educators with Tourette syndrome. Phenomenological research involves understanding what a particular experience is like for someone else. I also incorporated autoethnography in my study, which is my own personal narrative of my life and how living with Tourette syndrome has shaped my experiences.

This research is qualitative because qualitative research attempts to understand processes, concepts, and ideas, and is not measured in numbers. The purpose of my research is for the reader to be able to better understand what life is like for an educator with Tourette syndrome. Phenomenological research can go a long way in terms of teaching people about areas of life they have no way of experiencing for themselves.

As there is no literature on educators with Tourette syndrome, I want to be able to help people understand educators with disabilities, in this case Tourette syndrome. My research question was: How has having Tourette syndrome shaped educators' relationships in their personal and professional experiences? Some guiding questions were: How has having Tourette syndrome affected educators' relationships with their administrators? How has having Tourette syndrome affected educators' relationships with their colleagues? How has having Tourette syndrome affected educators' relationships with their students and their parents? Finally, how has Tourette shaped their own identity?

Implications for Practice

The number of people who participated in my study demonstrates that people with Tourette syndrome are indeed educators. The fact that my participants are from six different states shows that on a national level, there are educators with disabilities, specifically Tourette syndrome. Disability is no longer hidden and taboo; people with disabilities are coming out of the shadows to proclaim their citizenship (Longmore & Umansky, 2001). Longmore and Umansky comment, "If nothing else, disability has, it seems, at least won a place in the 'national conversation'" (2001, p.1). Hopefully, this study will encourage school districts to openly recruit educators with disabilities for employment. Not only do they possess characteristics of good teachers, they serve as role models to all students by showing others how people can overcome adversity in their lives.

Karp, Anderson, and Keller (1998) end with a message for school administrators considering hiring a person with disabilities as an educator. They state, "Educators with disabilities have been successful in schools but their presence in limited. You are in a key position to change the equation. We argue that the time is right for educators with disabilities to gain a greater presence in schools for they provide unique role models for children and add a depth to diversity in the work force that has yet to be fully exploited" (Karp, Anderson, & Keller, 1998, p. 277).

There is no way to put a statistic next to the number of schools that are not willing to hire educators with disabilities. Obviously, under the American with Disabilities Act (ADA), this is illegal. No administrator is going to admit to not hiring someone because he or she has a disability. An administrator is simply going to say, "We went with the best candidate." "I wondered—once again—if Tourette's would always keep me from leading a normal life. Would I forever be ejected from places other people enjoyed every day? Would I constantly be judged on my tics and twitches, rather than on who I was behind all that?" (Cohen, 2005, p. 93). What I am hoping to portray with this research is that educators with a disability are not a disability.

People have always had a fear of people who are different. In fact, this is the notion that dismodernism wraps itself around. Lennard Davis explains, "Rather than ignore the unstable nature of disability, rather than try to fix it, we should amplify that quality to distinguish it from other identity groups that have, as I have indicated, reached the limits of their own projects" (2002, p. 26). Dismodernism is the belief that difference is what we all have in common (Davis, 2002). Most of us will be disabled at some point in our lives (Davis, 2002). "Dependence, not individual independence, is the rule" (Davis, 2002, p. 26). The new catch phrase for dismodernism could be: form follows dysfunction (Davis, 2002).

Throughout history, people with disabilities have made other individuals who view themselves as "normal" uncomfortable (Longmore & Umansky, 2001). Longmore and Umansky write, "Americans often perceive disability—and therefore people with disabilities—as embodying that which Americans fear most: loss of independence, of autonomy, of control; in other words, subjection to fate" (2001, p. 7). As more and more people with disabilities are living their lives out of the shadows, why should people feel uncomfortable in the presence of people with disabilities? Perhaps this is because although we expect to find people with disabilities in medical institutions, we fail to look for them in everyday social settings (Longmore & Umansky, 2001).

Based on the data gathered from my study, these seven educators are just as competent and successful as any other educator. Additionally, they believe they are more understanding and sympathetic to students who have obstacles in their learning, or who do just no "get it" right away. These educators have pulled from their own experiences and found strengths from living with Tourette syndrome. They use these strengths to make them better educators.

Recommendations for Future Research

The participants in this study were all European Americans who self-identify as an educator with Tourette syndrome. The voice of educators with Tourette syndrome who do not identify as white is not heard in this research but needs to be. Studies of educators with another disability, such as Asperger's Syndrome, would also be beneficial.

Personal Implications

At the start of my doctoral studies, I had no idea I would ever contemplate writing on Tourette syndrome. Although I had made strides in coming to terms with my own disability, I was still extremely self-conscious. When it came down to it, I always worried about what other people thought. Even though it is common knowledge in my school district and my community that I have Tourette, I still try my hardest to suppress my tics. After writing a paper in my Social Context class about having Tourette syndrome, I started to play with the idea of centering my research around Tourette syndrome, but not without serious reservations.

When I finally decided to go ahead with the research, I was nervous and cautious. I knew the main contention in my research would be locating participants. I had no idea how many educators with Tourette syndrome were out there. What would be their incentive to contact me? Why would they want to share their story with me?

I was pleasantly surprised at the number of people who contacted me. As I carried out my research, I found these people were not only willing to share their experiences, but eager to have a voice in educating others about Tourette syndrome. My interviews with these people were enjoyable and engaging. It was so nice to be able to talk with others like me. Their stories mirrored mine; some of their experiences were so similar to my own. I had thought, felt, and sometimes even spoken the words that they used. As I listened to these people's stories, their triumphs and their struggles, I was inspired by their successes and moreover, their positive attitudes throughout. These people were determined not to let Tourette get the best of them. They worked tirelessly to become the competent, successful educators they are today. They successfully balanced the demands of being an educator along with the burden of being an educator with a disability. Moreover, they used the strengths they found in having Tourette to push them to become better teachers. They did not simply teach while having Tourette syndrome; they used the Tourette to make them better teachers. So many of them described themselves as more sympathetic, caring, compassionate, and open because they were educators with Tourette syndrome.

Not only were the participants enthusiastic about having a voice in order to educate others, they genuinely cared about the story I wanted to tell and the message I wanted to deliver. I received support and encouragement from them, the people whom without, this story would have never been told. All my participants let me know they thought I was doing great things and that they wanted to read my research once I had successfully finished it. Listening to their stories and the conversations we shared proved to be enlightening.

As I have said, the process of writing this book has been empowering for me. I want to note that although there may not be as many quotes in my data analysis from Stacy, she is the participant that I most nearly resemble, up until this school year. My first ten years of teaching, I have always tried my best to suppress my tics and not openly disclose that I have Tourette syndrome. Although it eventually became common knowledge among the faculty that I have Tourette, I never openly disclosed to my students. I was always too embarrassed and ashamed to talk about it openly.

In reference to disclosing, Oliva (2004) and the majority of her participants responded that they did not disclose and that they dreaded disclosing. Oliva (2004) felt this way herself for a long time. Many of Oliva's (2004) participants remember a sense of shame or embarrassment in telling people. Others in Oliva's (2004) survey remember feeling, "But I wasn't like THAT! I didn't want to be lumped with THEM" (p. 71). It is hard to be accepting of the fact that you have a disability and still maintain a healthy self-esteem. Many of Oliva's (2004) participants knew they should disclose, but experiences where disclosure brought no remedy or worsened the situation disinclined them to do so. Oliva (2004) comments how a lack of disclosure can stem from shame, yet more shame can result from experiences where disclosure accomplishes nothing.

Another sad article by Brock (2007) dealt with concealing disabilities. All but one of the participants with invisible disabilities reported concealing them during interviews, fearing that employment opportunities would be denied (Brock, 2007). Respondents who were diagnosed after employment concealed their disabilities, fearing that they would be perceived as less competent now that they were disabled (Brock, 2007). One participant stated, "I'm sure job discrimination exists. Consequently, I was not willing to lay out to others the real truth about my disability. Employers know they have to make adjustments, but the whole show changes then" (Brock, 2007, p. 11).

I sadly relate to these statements because in both of the school districts I have worked in, I concealed my Tourette syndrome during the interviews. I relate to what one respondent stated when it was explained, "I hadn't told my boss about my illness in the job interview. I wanted him to see me as a competent worker before he knew about my disability. Second, I wanted him and my colleagues to see me as a person before they saw me as a disease" (Brock, 2007, p. 12). Unfortunately, I know all too well what that feels like.

Another blow in Brock's (2007) article is the advice from a college administrator when he said, "Unless you plan to quit, don't tell. I hid my illness the first and second reoccurrence, but, my position was too high profile to hide the third time. It was the right decision each time.... Protect your privacy" (p. 12). This reminds me of my first year teaching at my current school district. During the first semester, my department chair called me into her office to ask how I was adjusting. She then said, "I legally cannot ask you anything about your health, but is everything okay?" I told her that I have movements or tics that were involuntary, but I tried to conceal them. Then, out of fear, I outright lied to her by saying, "It isn't Tourette's or anything like that."

One participant in Brock's (2007) article mentioned that she only disclosed her disability to her supervisor, and then she stated, "My supervisor didn't want people to know either" (p. 12). That brings me back to another sad experience in my teaching career. The semester before I began student teaching, I went to the school to meet my two cooperating teachers. I was prepared to be open and honest about my disability. I told them upfront that I had Tourette syndrome and asked for their advice about how to best explain this to my students. I wanted to play if off as it was not a big deal to me. They both advised me not to tell my students that I had Tourette because there was a student at that school who had a severe case of it, and he was very much an outcast and made fun of. They did not think me being associated with him would be good for my reputation.

That was hard on me because I had gone in with an open frame of mind, willing to disclose my disability. I know that my cooperating teachers were only thinking of my best interest, but it made it very difficult for me to try to suppress my tics all day long, for long periods of time without a break away from students.

Brock (2007) mentioned that only one respondent had positive advice about disclosing. She said, "Be honest, give your totally best effort, and expect honest fair treatment in return. Do not be afraid to stand up for yourself or worry about what others might say or think. My workplace doesn't penalize me for restricted health. It has been a good choice" (Brock, 2007, p. 12). I only wish I could have read those words before I started my student teaching career.

Brock (2007) mentions that all of the respondents who reported a visible disability and some whose disability was invisible felt the need to prove their worth and productivity by working harder than their co-workers. I can relate to this by taking on both paid and non-paid extracurricular activities at my current school district. I was a Renaissance breakfast sponsor for three years; this is a big reward for improving your grade point average or by having a high grade point average. I was also the Student Council sponsor for four years, which is a very demanding job with many activities throughout the school year.

Although this was a sad article for me to read, it did end on a positive note. Brock (2007) stated, "Although the ADA legislates inclusion, leadership, not legislation, molds societal attitudes. Educational leaders can influence attitudinal change by creating disability-friendly schools and modeling inclusion for educators with disabilities" (p. 13). I have been blessed at my current school district in working with principals, assistant principals, secretaries, guidance counselors, department chairs, and colleagues who have supported me when I have had students that wanted to make a production of my disability.

The support I receive at my school district is truly heartwarming.

This year, I thought long and hard about the first day with students. I felt a newfound sense of bravery after spending my summer vacation researching, interviewing others, and writing about Tourette syndrome. I felt that, although yes, it would be scary, I did not need to hide my disability from my students anymore. I decided I wanted to be more like Tracey, Mike, and Sue. I started with my class of juniors. I said on the first day, "How many of you have seen me around campus? Maybe I have subbed in one of your classes, or you have seen me in the tutoring room, or you have seen me in the hallway?" Most of them raised their hands. I then said, "How many of you have had a friend or a sibling who I have taught before?" About half of them raised their hands. I next said, "How many of you know I have Tourette syndrome?" Again, about half of them raised their hands. One student said, "What is Tourette syndrome?"

Over the course of the next ten minutes or so, I took what I had learned from Tracy, Mike, and Sue and explained what Tourette is. Like Tracey, I showed them some of the tics they may see me do, like jerking my arms or jerking my neck backward. I told them that the first couple of times they see me tic, they would probably be startled because it would catch them off guard. Then I said, "But I am willing to bet, after a few weeks, you won't even notice it anymore. You'll get used to me, you'll get used to my movements and the noises I make, and it won't even register to you."

Like Laura, my classroom is centered around the rule of respect. Respect yourselves, respect others, respect other people's property, respect any subs. I make it known when we go over the syllabus the first week of class that I work hard to make our classroom a safe environment. Like Tracey and Sue, I want everyone to feel safe to come to class and learn, and not be afraid of getting picked on or made fun of. I know that some students do not feel safe at home; some may not even have a home to go home to. I want them all to feel safe when they come into my classroom because only when one feels safe can learning begin. Respecting others and their differences is integral to this process.

Like Tracey and Mike, I gave the students a question and answer period to ask about Tourette syndrome. Similar to their experiences, I found that after a few initial questions about Tourette syndrome, my students were much more interested in hearing about the different universities I have attended and degrees I have received and the fact that I am writing a book over 200 pages long than they were about the fact that I have Tourette syndrome. Although I am only four weeks into the new school year, I have found how true it is that once you educate children, they are extremely accepting.

With one of my senior classes, we discussed discrimination at the beginning of the school year. The first current events packet that I handed out to them was on Tourette syndrome. Before we read it, I talked about how I have been discriminated against at various times in my life because of the fact that I have Tourette syndrome. We talked about how discrimination is not right nor is it fair, but it is a reality. After reading about what Tourette syndrome is, along with an article about James Durbin, the *American Idol* contestant with Tourette syndrome, as well as a newspaper article from an out of state newspaper that Tracey sent me two months after we finished our interviews, we talked about what it feels like to be discriminated against. This class discussion turned into our first writing assignment of the year: a time when we were discriminated against or treated unfairly at some point in our lives. I prefaced this with the statement that I hope none of them have ever been discriminated against before, but in reality, I know it happens. I told them if they were lucky enough never to have experienced discrimination before, then to write about a time when someone they know was treated unfairly, or write about an event that they saw on the news or read about somewhere.

The essays I received were phenomenal. These young adults talked about how they had been treated unfairly in the past because of their ethnicity or their religion. Others wrote about being treated unfairly because they were overweight. Another student wrote about being discriminated against because she was bisexual. Although we did not share these stories in class, reading them reiterated the point I made to them that, "Everyone has something." There is no need to make a big ordeal about something because everyone has something they are dealing with. It could be a death in the family or a learning disability, or it could be something more noticeable like my Tourette syndrome, but we are all dealing with something. Perseverance is the key. It is okay to struggle, as long as you keep on keeping on.

I would not say that I openly disclose one hundred percent of the time. I would definitely not say that I have overcome Tourette. However, I am not quitting. I continue working every day; I try to make people more knowledgeable about Tourette, and I try to be more open to disclosing about my disability every day. I continue to work and try. And that is the key to overcoming adversity. It is the mantra of never say die. I will not let Tourette syndrome get the best of me. I will not let Tourette syndrome beat me.

This entire research process, from selecting a topic, to writing my story and listening to and writing my participants' stories proved to indeed be empowering. I found myself initiating conversations with colleagues at work and with friends about my research. I would bravely tell people how I had always been too insecure to discuss my Tourette with others and how this whole event had been a growing process for me. I hope this research shows people, not just with Tourette syndrome but with any disability, that having a disability is not a disability. Life may not always be easy, but we persevere. We did not choose to have a disability. This life chose us. However, anything you want to do can be achieved. In fact, if you can take your disability and pull from the strengths it gives you, you will be a better person for it. I know I am.

218

References

American Psychiatric Association. (1994). Diagnostic and statistical manual of mental disorders (4th ed.). Washington, DC: Author.

Anderson, R.J. (1998). Attitudes toward educators with disabilities. In R.J. Anderson, C.E. Keller, & J.M. Karp (Eds.), *Enhancing diversity: Educators with disabilities.* Washington, DC: Gallaudet University Press.

Brock, B.A. (2007). The workplace experience of educators with disabilities: Insights for school leaders. *Educational Considerations, 34(2),* 9-14.

Cohen, B., & Wysocky, L. (2005). *Front of the class: How tourette syndrome made me the teacher I never had.* New York: St. Martin's Griffin.

Davis, L. J. (2002). *Bending over backwards: Disability, dismodernism, and other difficult positions.* New York, NY: New York University Press.

Harrell, C. (2007, October). Why are districts hesitant towards hiring teachers with disabilities. *Americans with Disabilities.* Retrieved June 10, 2009, from http://www.associatedcontent.com/article/407654/why_are_distri cts_hesitiant_towards.html?cat=4

Hehir, T. (2005). *New directions in special education: Eliminating ableism in policy and practice.* Cambridge, MA. Harvard Education Press.

Jackson, E.M. (2002). Virginia educators with disabilities survey results. *Virginia Board for People with Disabilities.* Retrieved June 10, 2009, from http://www.vaboard.org/policyfellowship.htm

Karp, J.M., & Keller, C.E. (1998). Preparation and employment experiences of educators with disabilities. In R.J. Anderson, C.E. Keller, & J.M. Karp (Eds.), *Enhancing diversity: Educators with disabilities.* Washington, DC: Gallaudet University Press.

Kumari Campbell, F.A. (2008). Exploring internalized ableism using critical race theory. *Disability and Society, 23(2),* 151-162.

Kumari Campbell, F. (2009). *Contours of ableism: The production of disability and abledness.* Great Britain: Palgrave Macmillan.

Longmore, P.K., & Umansky, L. Disability history: From the margins to the mainstream. In P.K. Longmore & L. Umansky (Eds.), *The new disability history: American perspectives* (pp. 1-29). New York, NY: New York University Press.

Marks, D. (1999). *Disability: Controversial debates and psychosocial perspectives.* London: Rutledge.

Massey, D.S. (2007). *Categorically Unequal: The American stratification system.* New York, NY: Russell Sage Foundation.

McKay, G. (2001). Back to school 2001: Disabilities no handicap as teachers rise above physical problems to do classroom jobs. *PG News.* Retrieved June 10, 2009, from http://www.post-gazette.com/regionstate/20010827disabledschooltworeg2p2.asp

Merriam, S. B. (2009). *Qualitative research: A guide to design and implementation.* San Francisco, CA: Jossey-Bass.

Morrison, J. (1995). DSM-IV made easy: The clinician's guide to diagnoses. New York, NY: Guilford Press.

Oliva, G.A. (2004). *Alone in the mainstream: A deaf woman remembers public school.* Washington, DC: Gallaudet University Press.

Patton, M.Q. (2002). *Qualitative research and evaluation methods.* Thousand Oaks, CA: Sage Publications.

Rosenwasser, P. (2000). Tool for transformation: Co-operative inquiry as a process for healing from internalized oppression. Paper presented at the Adult Education Research Conference (AERC), June 2-4, in British Columbia. http://www.edst.edu.ubc.ca/aerc/2000/rosenwasserpl-final.PDF

Seidman, I. (2006). *Interviewing as qualitative research: A guide for researchers in education and the social sciences.* New York, NY: Teachers College Press.

Shapiro, J.P. (1993). *No pity: People with disabilities forging a new civil rights movement.* New York, NY: Three Rivers Press.

Wills, D.K. (2007). The advantage of the disadvantage: Teachers with disabilities are not a handicap. *Edutopia.* Retrieved June 10, 2009, from http://www.edutopia.org/disabled-teachers

Wolcott, H.F. (2010). *Ethnography lessons: A primer.* Walnut Creek, CA: Left Coat Press.

NEXT

How can you empower educators with disabilities and people with Tourette syndrome? How can you encourage others to read this book?

1. Write a review on Amazon (and on your blog or Facebook page)
2. Give a copy of this book to a friend
3. Get an autographed copy of the book
4. Order books in bulk (discount based on quantity) to use with a group (email quantity to obtain quote)
5. Get involved with an organization that makes a difference, such as the Tourette Syndrome Association

Need more information on any of these possibilities? Send an email to the publisher at: jkspress@gmail.com.

Manufactured by Amazon.ca
Bolton, ON